EASY KETO DIET FOR BEGINNERS

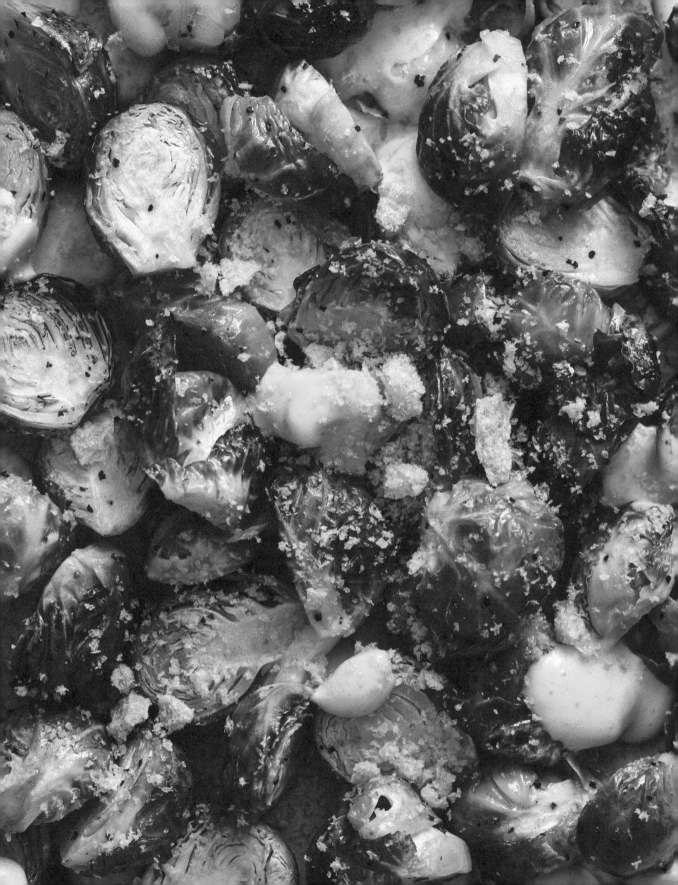

EASY KETO DIET FOR BEGINNERS

A Complete Guide to Kick-Start the Ketogenic Lifestyle

COMPILED BY FRANK CAMPANELLA

ROCKRIDGE PRESS

For general information on our other products and services or to obtain technical support, please contact our Customer Care Department within the United States at (866) 744-2665, or outside the United States at (510) 253-0500.

Rockridge Press publishes its books in a variety of electronic and print formats. Some content that appears in print may not be available in electronic books, and vice versa.

TRADEMARKS: Rockridge Press and the Rockridge Press logo are trademarks or registered trademarks of Callisto Media Inc. and/or its affiliates, in the United States and other countries, and may not be used without written permission. All other trademarks are the property of their respective owners. Rockridge Press is not associated with any product or vendor mentioned in this book.

Interior and Cover Designer: Karmen Lizzul
Art Producer: Meg Baggott
Editor: Reina Glenn
Production Editor: Jenna Dutton
Production Manager: Martin Worthington

Cover photo ©2021 Hélène Dujardin. Food styling by Anna Hampton.

Alicia Cho, ii, x, 50; Lauren Flippen, v, 34, 166; Biz Jones, vi; 52, 86, 99, 100, 136, 190; Evi Abeler, xii, 20, 154; Nadine Greeff, 49; Darren Muir, 68; Hélène Dujardin, 116, 178. Illustrations, Shutterstock.

Author photo courtesy of Amanda Caldwell

Paperback ISBN: 978-1-63807-032-0
eBook ISBN: 978-1-63807-147-1

R1

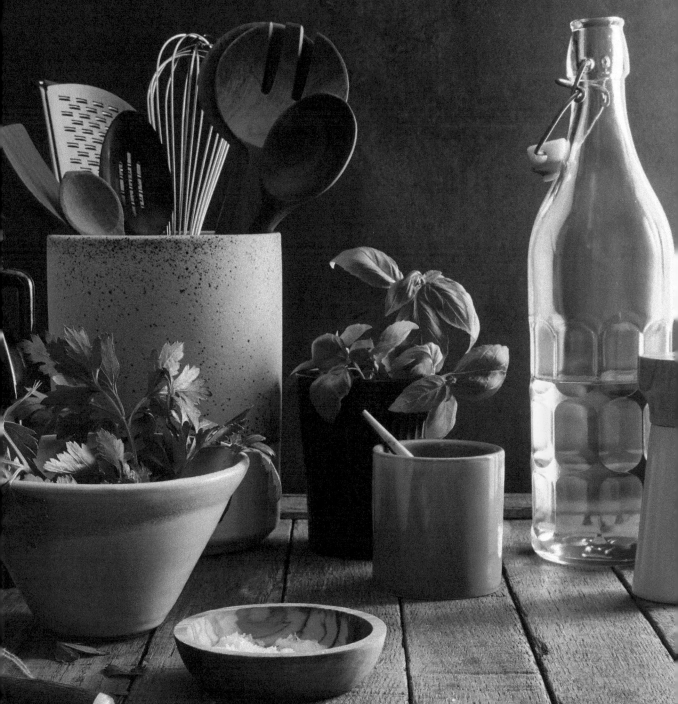

THANK YOU TO MY FRIENDS AND FAMILY, WHO HAVE ALWAYS SUPPORTED ME THROUGHOUT MY CAREER AND BEYOND. I PROMISE TO INVITE YOU TO THE LAKE HOUSE . . . ONCE IT'S BUILT.

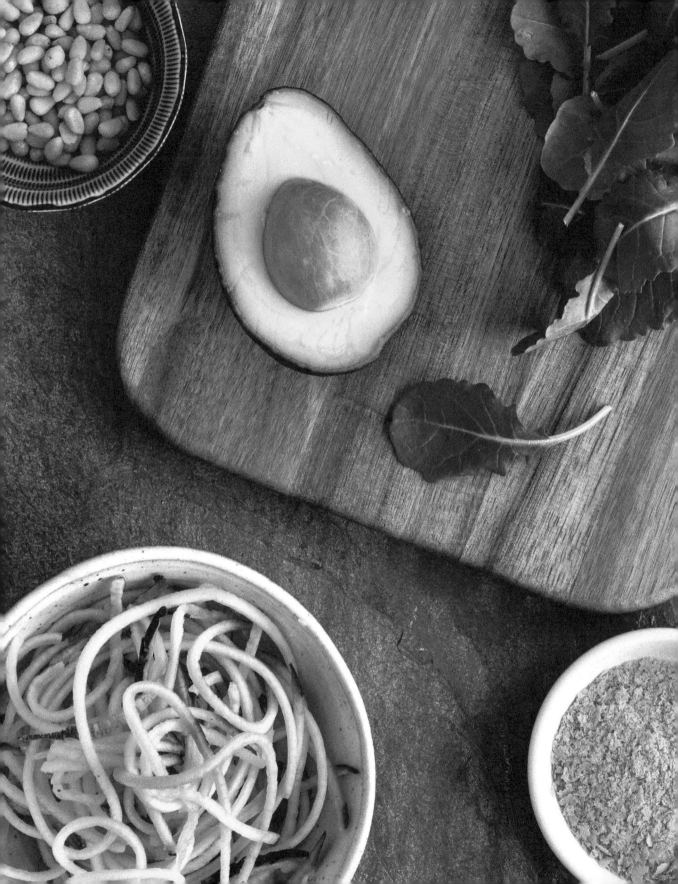

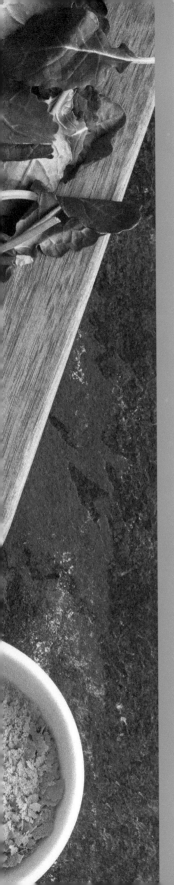

CONTENTS

INTRODUCTION

My keto journey started about four years ago, when I found myself morbidly obese and unable to live the life that I wanted. I had tried just about every diet with little to no success. Discouraged by the lack of results, I was convinced I just couldn't lose weight. Then things got even worse when I found myself in the hospital, fighting for my life against an infection. Things had to change, but I didn't know where to begin. After a chance conversation with a trainer, I discovered a new approach to eating known as the ketogenic diet.

As a chef, I already knew how to cook, but instead of the carb-heavy ingredients I was used to, I began to concentrate on whole foods that were high in protein and low in carbs. When the weight began to come off, I was invigorated with confidence. I had (finally!) found a lifestyle that I could stick to long-term. I was hooked on the fresh veggies, high-quality protein, and even sugar-free baked goods for an occasional treat. I started posting recipes on social media, which soon became a website, and now I create and share my ketogenic and low-carb recipes full time with people all over the world.

Though I am still on my journey to reach my goal weight, I am able to share my experiences with others and help them avoid the mistakes I made when starting on the ketogenic diet. Today, I am able to enjoy almost all the cuisines and foods I used to love—but in a healthier way, using higher-quality ingredients. My world has opened up with opportunities that four years ago I would never have thought possible. I hope this book can give you the building blocks to reach your own health and fitness goals to live your best life.

Whether you want to lose 20 pounds or 200, the ketogenic diet is a lifestyle that has endless health benefits, including giving you better energy to get active. This book will teach you the foundation of the ketogenic diet and how to navigate the ups and downs of the journey. You will learn which foods to incorporate into your diet and which to limit or avoid. Make sure to consult with your doctor before making major lifestyle changes.

To make starting (and sticking to) the diet as easy as possible, follow this book's 4-Week Meal Plan (page 35). Along with recipes that are simple and approachable without sacrificing flavor, the plan provides shopping lists and nutritional information to help keep you on track. Both in and outside of the meal plan, the recipes in this book are familiar favorites reimagined in a healthier way. Mostly, they feature ingredients that you'll commonly find in grocery stores, as well as a few new keto-specific items that will quickly become staples in your pantry.

Any lifestyle change can seem scary at first, but know that this decision to invest in yourself is worthy of celebration. We only get one body and one life, so I'm really glad you've decided to make the most of this opportunity. I've been where you are now and I'm rooting for your success. You've got this!

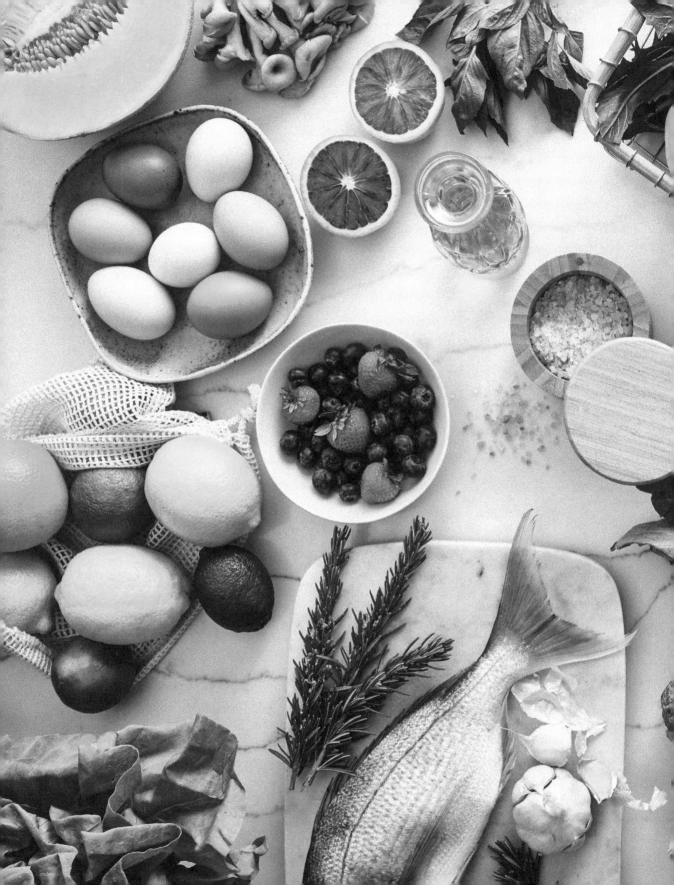

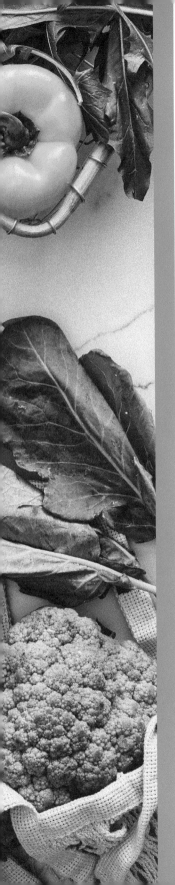

PART ONE

Welcome to Keto

In part 1, we will go over the basics, including what the ketogenic diet is and how to get the most out of it. We'll discuss the advantages of being in ketosis and how to calculate your macros for optimized health. You'll also learn about how your glucose levels can affect your body's hunger signals and energy levels.

Before you overhaul your pantry, it's important to familiarize yourself with the ingredients you will need to look for and those you should avoid. You will learn about different types of hidden sugars that are found in common foods, and which healthier alternatives to use. We will also discuss what you can do to prepare for your new lifestyle and how to avoid common pitfalls.

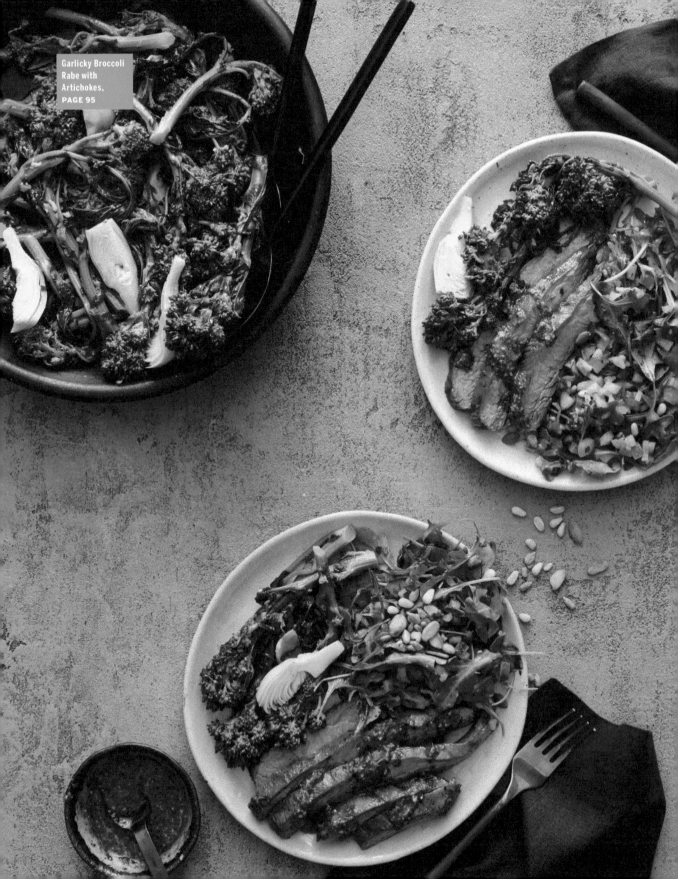

Garlicky Broccoli Rabe with Artichokes, PAGE 95

CHAPTER 1

Keto 101

Let's start at the beginning. What is the ketogenic diet, and why does it work? In this chapter, you'll learn how your body can use fat as a fuel source instead of sugar, and why that equals more energy and less hunger throughout the day. The ketogenic diet really can jump-start a healthier lifestyle. Let's dive in.

HOW THE KETOGENIC DIET WORKS

Did you know that your body has two fuel sources?

The first source is **glucose**. Your body creates glucose from the carbohydrates (carbs) you eat in grains, breads, pastas, sugar, and starches, to name a few. Glucose is a readily available fuel source that your body can use for energy, but it is not long lasting, and the process of converting carbs to glucose sends your blood sugar on a roller-coaster ride (a "glu-coaster," if you will).

Here is how it works:

1. After you consume carbohydrates (think refined grains and sugars), your body begins to digest them into glucose.

2. This process of converting carbs to glucose causes a spike in your blood sugar and gives you a temporary energy boost (this is where the term "sugar high" comes from).

3. In response to this aggressive blood sugar spike (and because a glucose overdose in your bloodstream can be toxic), your body reacts by signaling the pancreas to release the hormone insulin, which acts to remove the excess glucose from your bloodstream.

4. The released insulin works swiftly to transport the glucose out of your bloodstream to burn as fuel and then puts the rest in storage (more on this in a minute).

5. As the insulin removes the glucose from your bloodstream, your blood sugar subsequently drops, your energy level declines, and you feel hungry again.

6. So you eat more carbs, and the cycle begins again . . .

This process explains why most people get an afternoon energy crash around 3:00 p.m. and start craving sweets or candy. It is not your lack of willpower that causes these cravings. It is your body saying, "Hey! My blood sugar is low and I need more energy—give me carbs now!"

If being on the never-ending glu-coaster isn't bad enough, there's one more important fact you should know. Depending on how much energy you need (which is based primarily on your physical activity level), you burn that specific amount of glucose and the rest gets stored in your body. Some of the excess glucose is converted into glycogen and stored in your liver and muscle tissues for future use. But the remaining glucose that your body didn't use is stored as fat in the form of triglycerides. That's right: Your body stores the excess glucose in your fat cells and essentially forgets about it.

Then, of course, the whole cycle starts again. You eat more carbs at your next meal, you jump on the glu-coaster, your body uses what it needs for energy and stores the rest as fat. And those fat cells keep piling up. This is the reason you gain weight.

But there's good news! Your body has another fuel source: **ketones**.

Ketones are amazing little energy pods your body creates from stored fat. Yes, you heard me correctly: You can turn those stored fat cells into energy. And not just any kind of energy—energy that is long-lasting and consistent, meaning no afternoon crashes. When you use ketones for energy, your body is using its own stored fat as fuel. Thus, you start losing weight. Brilliant, right?

The goal of the ketogenic diet is to capitalize on all this by training your body to start burning ketones for energy instead of glucose. This phenomenon is called ketosis. When your body is in a state of ketosis, it becomes a literal fat-burning machine.

So to summarize, these are the basics:

What is a ketogenic diet? It is a low-carb, moderate-protein, high-fat diet designed to exhaust glucose levels and prompt the body to provide an alternative source of energy to the brain. These alternative energy sources are called ketones, which are produced by the liver using stored fat.

What is ketosis? When the body takes stored fat through the liver and produces ketones (small molecules used as fuel throughout the body), it is called ketosis.

Why do you want to be in ketosis? Ketosis is the way for humans to operate most efficiently and can lead to numerous benefits such as weight loss, increased energy, improved focus, better sleep, clearer skin, strength gain, reduced appetite, better digestion, and balanced mood, to name a few.

What to Expect on the Keto Diet

1. **Fewer cravings.** Because it eliminates blood sugar crashes, a ketogenic diet will gradually decrease your desire for unhealthy foods, such as cake or donuts. Even when you do occasionally indulge, a bite or two will be enough, as your body will no longer rely on those carbs as sources of energy.

2. **Reduced appetite.** Not only will eating ketogenically kill your cravings for carbs, it will decrease your appetite as well because carbs stimulate your appetite. Eating a low-carb diet keeps your appetite in check so you eat fewer calories and lose weight naturally. Write down what you eat for a few days. Don't go hungry, but see what you eat. I'll bet you'll be surprised by how few calories you take in.

3. **Rapid weight loss—especially in the beginning.** It will be mostly water weight that you lose at the beginning, because your body holds onto excess water when you eat too many carbs. But even after the initial drop, you'll lose weight faster with keto than you will with other diets—particularly low-fat diets—due to ketosis fat burning. If you maintain the lifestyle, you'll keep it off longer, too.

4. **Full-fat ingredients.** Do not, under any circumstances, eat low-fat or reduced-fat anything. Eat butter. Eat full-fat cheese and milk. Fry your eggs in lard. Eating a diet that is 70 percent fat, 25 percent protein, and only 15 percent carbs will also raise your HDL (good) cholesterol and decrease your triglycerides, according to a 2003 study in the *Journal of Pediatrics*.

5. **Decreased risk for metabolic syndrome, high blood pressure, high blood sugar, and type 2 diabetes.** High blood sugar alone isn't type 2 diabetes; however, prolonged exposure to high blood sugar can cause your pancreas to reduce its production of insulin, causing type 2 diabetes. Basically, in type 2 diabetes, your body becomes desensitized to the presence of sugar. If you have these conditions already, they may decrease or disappear altogether on a keto diet.

6. **More muscle, less fat.** By consuming muscle meat and protein, you are building muscle—and therefore increasing your metabolism. Protein is anabolic (promotes metabolic activity) and used for building new cells, such as muscle. Muscles require more energy to move, so just by building more muscle mass, you are burning more energy and raising your metabolism. According to McKinley Health Center at the University of Illinois at Urbana-Champaign, some people have genetics to thank for having higher metabolic rates than others, but it's important to consider muscle mass when determining your basal metabolic rate (BMR). Muscle is more active and demands more energy than fat, so if you have a higher percentage of muscle compared to fat, you will have a higher BMR.

7. **Increased gut health.** We all hear about probiotics and improving the bacteria in our gut, but how can eating ketogenically help with that? Sugars and processed foods cause inflammation in your intestinal tract. When you combine carbs, processed foods, and stress, tiny perforations form in your intestinal walls, and waste products and digestive acids that shouldn't leave your intestinal tract end up leaking out. According to Harvard Health Publications, the rush of blood sugar you get when eating a meal or snack of highly refined carbohydrates (white bread, white rice, French fries, sugar-laden soda, etc.) increases your level of inflammatory messengers called cytokines.

GETTING INTO KETOSIS

The ketogenic diet is simple in its implementation (goal: stay in ketosis); however, the path can be different for each person. Everyone begins at 20 net carbohydrates and then, over time, determines how many carbs they can consume without being kicked out of ketosis. It's up to each of us to learn what our personal "kick out" point is and stay below it.

How do you know if you are in ketosis? Simple: keto sticks. Tubes of these thin test strips are available at your local pharmacy. Simply urinate on a stick to find out if you're in or out of ketosis. If the stick turns light pink, you're out of ketosis; any shade of purple means you're in. Note that a darker shade of purple does not indicate "better" ketosis—it matters only if you are in or out, burning fat or not. There aren't tiers or levels you need to reach. However, if you're diabetic, you run the risk of a condition called "ketoacidosis" on a ketogenic diet. Be sure to talk with your doctor about the diet; they will likely recommend using keto sticks and making sure you stay in the light purple range.

To calculate net carbohydrates, take the number of carbs you consume and subtract the number of fiber grams consumed. This is the number you'll use to track your daily total. When food is high in fiber, such as coconut, you can eat more of it even if the carbohydrate numbers look a little scary. Some people on the keto diet find that paying attention to macros (or daily percentages of foods that fall into the three main macronutrient categories: carbohydrates, proteins, and fat) is helpful for keeping track of their weight loss, and other people use them for medical reasons. If you don't have any medical reasons to stick to certain percentages, then a good daily starting point for the ketogenic diet is 5 percent carbs, 20 percent proteins, and 75 percent fats. If this doesn't keep you in ketosis, try 5 percent carbs, 15 percent proteins, and 80 percent fats. (To help you, there are macro percentages listed in each of the upcoming recipes.)

Ultimately, it's up to you to find a balance that works. There are hundreds of calculators online that you can use to input your stats—weight, height, sex, weight goal, and so on—and the calculator will tell you what is supposed to be the ideal macro for you. The amount of carbs (which generally should come from vegetables) or fats that will create ketosis in the body varies for different people. It is certainly not an exact science. See Calculating Your Ratios (page 7) for a good starting place.

Calculating Your Ratios

Your *macronutrient ratio* consists of the amounts of fat, protein, and carbs that you should consume daily in relation to one another. For example, the Bacon-Wrapped Barbecue Turkey Meatballs (page 124) has a macronutrient breakdown of Fat 59% / Protein 30% / Carbs 11%. Its fat-to-protein ratio is 2:1, meaning there are 2 grams of fat for every 1 gram of protein.

Two factors that influence your macronutrient level are lean mass weight (what you weigh without any fat) and activity level. Here are some examples of the latter:

→ **SEDENTARY:** Most office jobs, very little or no exercise (light walking)

→ **LIGHTLY ACTIVE:** One to three times a week, light exercise such as light cardio (walking, light cycling)

→ **MODERATELY ACTIVE:** Three to five times a week (moderate cardio and muscle training)

→ **VERY ACTIVE:** Five or more times a week (hard exercise, intense cardio and muscle training at fitness level)

→ **ATHLETES/BODYBUILDERS:** Daily exercise at professional level (high-intensity exercise)

Following is a basic formula to help you work out your macronutrient ratio. Say you weigh 160 pounds and have 30 percent body fat. Your lean mass weight would be calculated as follows:

160 pounds − 30% (48 pounds) = 112 pounds

Multiply the result by 0.6 to determine the minimum grams of protein you should consume:

112 × 0.6 = 67 g protein

Multiply the first result by 1 to determine the maximum grams of protein you should consume:

112 × 1 = 112 g protein

Therefore, your daily protein intake should be between 67 and 112 grams.

THE GUIDELINES

Other than maintaining a caloric deficit, sticking to your macros is one of the biggest keys to success with the ketogenic diet. Staying hydrated and incorporating electrolytes into your routine are also extremely important for overall health. Keep track of your macros and make adjustments to find the balance that works best for you.

Stick to your macros. The daily 5/20/75 ratio is worth sticking to because it works. Too many carbs and you won't burn fat. Too much protein and it won't burn off if you don't use it. Not enough fat and you won't be full. All these problems add up to less energy. The recommended ratio allows for a holistic approach to ketosis.

Keep your electrolytes up. Electrolytes are the minerals in your blood that keep you hydrated and allow your nerves and muscles to work properly in balance. By producing ketones, you'll be flushing out more electrolytes than usual. This means you should increase your salt intake while following keto because your body won't hang onto sodium the way it used to. Most ketoers do this by drinking chicken broth or bouillon daily, especially in the first few weeks of ketosis while the body is adjusting. If you feel achy in the first week on keto while going through carbohydrate withdrawal, bouillon helps. Many ketoers use magnesium supplements as well.

Drink lots of water. Drinking two to three liters of water every day will make your body feel clean, full, and hydrated; keep your bowels moving; and help you lose weight faster if that's your goal.

Keep track of what you eat. Measuring what you eat turns any diet into a game. Use apps such as MyFitnessPal to track your meals and measure your macros at the end of the day. There's also an app called Quip that you can use to make shopping lists. It includes check marks that allow you to reuse your shopping list every week.

Eat your calories. Don't try to do a low-calorie ketogenic diet, or you'll end up without any fuel. Fat is your new fuel. Without it, you'll not only be hungry, but you also won't lose weight. Many ketoers eat 1,800 calories or more per day and find that eating less than that actually makes them stop losing weight. But don't over-indulge, either. You likely won't lose weight eating 5,000 calories a day. The good news is that you won't be hungry enough to eat that much anyway!

Stock up on healthy fats. There are plenty of good fats out there, such as ghee, which is lactose- and casein-free clarified butter that's high in anti-inflammatory, omega-3 fatty acids. For times when you run out of this magical golden buttery oil, keep a backup of coconut oil and olive oil. Avoid processed oils such as vegetable, sunflower seed, soybean, and corn—they are high in inflammatory omega-6s, which in turn destroy the healthy omega-3s in your body.

Invest in certified organic, grass-fed, and free-range products. Now that your diet is exchanging highly refined carbohydrates for mostly fats and proteins, you'll want to pay extra-special attention to the quality of those ingredients.

Stick to real food, not low-carb products. If you check the label of most low-carb products, unless they're also paleo products, you'll be shocked to find that their ingredients include unpronounceable chemical additives. You can control what goes into your body by making your own meals and sticking to whole foods.

Clean vs. Dirty Keto?

This book loosely follows the "clean" version of keto, which is the healthiest way to get into ketosis and burn fat instead of carbs. There's another version—"dirty" keto—that can do the same thing. So, what's the difference?

Clean keto focuses on eating high-quality, minimally processed or preserved whole foods to achieve ketosis. Grass-fed beef, free-range eggs, and organic vegetables are staples of a clean keto diet. Use them whenever possible, as your budget allows. On the other hand, followers of dirty keto can eat whatever they want to reach ketosis, as long as they maintain macro percentages of 70 to 75 percent fat, 20 to 25 percent protein, and 5 to 10 percent carbs. Processed foods are allowed in dirty keto, as are foods from favorite fast food restaurants. Keto-friendly versions of foods such as cookies, cakes, and chips are also fine on a dirty keto diet.

For people new to the ketogenic lifestyle, the dirty keto diet can be a real lifesaver, making a daunting diet feel a lot more achievable because you don't have to rely on cooking every single meal. Many people have had great success following the keto diet while still eating at some of their favorite restaurants and taking the edge off their cravings with keto-friendly snacks.

However, over time, the dirty keto diet can backfire on some people. By continuing to eat keto-friendly versions of cookies and chips, they never break the habit of eating junk food. Additives such as antibiotics, pesticides, and preservatives can slow the body's healing process. Plus, many people find that the processed ingredients in keto-friendly snacks, such as sugar alcohols and chemicals, start to have a negative effect on their bodies and even kick them out of ketosis.

As in all good things, moderation is key. In the beginning, dirty keto isn't bad and can make the transition to a low-carb diet much easier (you'll notice that some recipes in this book call for sugar substitutes and processed meats—this is to help you as a beginner). In the long run, a successful ketogenic lifestyle is all about an escalation: making good, better, and then the best choices.

FOODS TO LOVE, LIMIT, AND AVOID

The foods we eat on a keto diet can be divided into three categories: love, limit, and avoid. But even the foods you should avoid have healthier alternatives, so you won't be going without. Having these categories in your head will make it easier to shop for foods that will provide solid nutrition throughout your journey.

Foods to Love

Keto isn't as restrictive as you might think. Yes, you need to eliminate most carbs, but there's a long list of delicious, nutritious foods to take their place. Focus on the following categories when structuring your plates.

FATS AND OILS

Superstar: extra-virgin olive oil. Olive oil is high in monounsaturated fat, contains the powerful antioxidant oleuropein, and has been shown in numerous studies to improve heart-disease risk markers. Other fats and oils to eat include:

→ Avocado oil
→ Butter
→ Coconut oil
→ Egg yolks
→ Ghee
→ Lard

→ Macadamia nut oil
→ MCT oil
→ Organic, unrefined red palm oil

→ Sesame oil
→ Tallow (fat from sheep and cattle)
→ Walnut oil

NUTS AND SEEDS

Superstar: macadamia nuts. Of all the nuts, macadamia has the lowest omega-6-to-omega-3 ratio. Researchers believe that lowering this ratio can help lower inflammation and obesity risk. Other nuts and seeds to eat include:

→ Almonds

→ Brazil nuts

→ Cashews

→ Coconut meat (shredded or whole)

→ Hazelnuts

→ Nut butter (made with any of the nuts listed)

→ Pecans

→ Pistachios

→ Pumpkin seeds

→ Sunflower seeds

→ Tahini (sesame seed paste)

→ Walnuts

PROTEINS

Superstar: eggs. The egg is the ideal keto food: high-fat, medium protein, and very low-carb. Plus, egg yolks are rich in important nutrients such as choline and vitamin A. Other proteins to eat include:

→ Beef

→ Collagen protein powder

→ Fish (includes cod, mackerel, mahi mahi, red snapper, salmon, and tuna)

→ Lamb

→ Organ meats (includes heart, kidney, and liver)

→ Pork

→ Poultry (includes chicken, duck, and turkey)

→ Shellfish (includes clams, lobster, oysters, and shrimp)

→ Vegan protein options (includes hemp protein, pea protein, tempeh, tofu, and vegan cheese)

→ Whey protein powder

DAIRY PRODUCTS

Superstar: butter. Butter is high in vitamins A, D, and K, as well as the anti-inflammatory compound butyrate. Get your butter from pasture-raised cows for maximum nutrition. Other dairy products to eat include:

→ Cheese (includes Brie, cream cheese, feta, goat, Gouda, mozzarella, and Parmesan)

→ Heavy cream

→ Whole milk

→ Yogurt

Note: *Many folks don't react well to the lactose (milk sugar) or casein (milk protein) in these foods. If you're one of these people, use almond and coconut products in recipes calling for dairy.*

NONSTARCHY VEGETABLES

Superstar: kale. Kale is rich in vitamin K, the antioxidants lutein and zeaxanthin, and isothiocyanates—compounds with promising anticancer effects. Other nonstarchy vegetables to eat include:

→ Arugula

→ Asparagus

→ Bok choy

→ Broccoli

→ Brussels sprouts

→ Cabbage

→ Cauliflower

→ Mushrooms

→ Romaine lettuce

→ Spinach

→ Watercress

Note: *This list isn't comprehensive because there are simply too many vegetables to name. As a general rule, look for vegetables with under 5 grams of net carbs per serving (you want to stay under about 20 grams of net carbs per day).*

FLAVORINGS AND SWEETENERS

Superstar: erythritol. Noncaloric and a potent antioxidant, erythritol doesn't raise blood sugar and insulin levels like most other sweeteners do. Other sweeteners and flavorings to eat include:

→ Allulose
→ Brown sugar replacement
→ Cocoa powder
→ Monk fruit
→ Stevia
→ Vanilla extract

BEVERAGES

Superstar: green tea. Compounds in green tea called catechins may help stimulate weight loss by increasing metabolic rate. Other beverages to drink include:

→ Almond milk
→ Black tea
→ Broth
→ Coffee
→ Hemp milk
→ Herbal tea
→ Lemon juice
→ Sparkling water

Foods to Limit

Enjoy the following foods in moderation on the keto diet.

Alcohol: Alcohol won't help your keto goals, but the occasional serving of wine or hard alcohol (both low-carb) should be fine. Strive to avoid concoctions with added sugar, though.

Avocados: Technically a fruit, avocados are high in fiber, monounsaturated fat, and vitamin E, but also contain 12 grams of carbs. Limit to one per day.

Berries (includes blueberries, raspberries, cranberries, and blackberries): These fruits are low in sugar and high in antioxidants. You can have a few berries, but keep portions small to limit carbs.

Dark chocolate: Shoot for at least 85 percent cacao bars with minimal added sugar.

Processed meats (includes ham, prosciutto, hot dogs, lunch meats, and pepperoni): These meats are okay in moderation, but be strict about label reading—they can contain added sugar, artificial ingredients, and preservatives. Look for all-natural, organic, no-sugar-added versions of these items and limit consumption to a few times per week.

Tomatoes: Though high in the antioxidant lutein, tomatoes also have about 5 grams of carbs each.

Turnips and carrots: Though most root vegetables are too starchy for the keto diet, turnips and carrots have a relatively lower amount of carbs and are okay in small amounts.

Foods to Eliminate

Get the donation bag ready. Here are the foods that don't belong in your keto kitchen.

GRAINS

Why avoid? Grains contain too many carbs for keto. Grains also contain compounds such as gluten, phytic acid, and lectins that damage the gut and block nutrient absorption. Examples include:

- → Barley
- → Bread
- → Corn
- → Millet
- → Oats
- → Pasta
- → Quinoa
- → Rice
- → Rye

STARCHY VEGETABLES

Why avoid? These foods aren't unhealthy per se, but they'll spike insulin and keep you from entering ketosis. Examples include:

- → Beets
- → Parsnips
- → Potatoes
- → Sweet potatoes

SUGARY FRUITS

Why avoid? Except for berries, tomatoes, avocados, lemons, and limes, most fruits are too high in fructose (sugar) to make the keto cut. Examples include:

- → Apples
- → Bananas
- → Cherries
- → Grapes
- → Kiwi fruit
- → Melon (all types)
- → Oranges
- → Peaches
- → Plums

ANYTHING WITH ADDED SUGAR

Why avoid? Sugar raises insulin levels and prevents fat-burning. In other words, sugar is the nemesis of ketosis. Examples include:

- → Candy
- → Cookies
- → Crackers
- → Granola bars
- → Juice
- → Salad dressing
- → Soda
- → Tomato sauce

> **Pro tip:** *To avoid refined sugar, shop the periphery of the grocery store. If it comes in a package, there's probably sugar in it.*

INDUSTRIAL SEED OILS

Why avoid? These vegetable oils are high in the inflammatory omega-6 fat linoleic acid. Researchers believe that excessive linoleic acid consumption is partly responsible for the American obesity epidemic. Examples include:

- → Canola oil
- → Corn oil
- → Cottonseed oil
- → Peanut oil
- → Safflower oil
- → Soybean oil
- → Sunflower oil

> **Pro tip:** *Avoid cooking with these unstable oils. They oxidize when heated, forming compounds called oxidized lipids, which drive the progression of heart disease.*

ARTIFICIAL SWEETENERS

Why avoid? A study published in the journal *Diabetes Care* found that drinking just one artificially sweetened soda per day is associated with a 67 percent higher risk of type 2 diabetes. Examples include:

- → Acesulfame potassium
- → Aspartame
- → Saccharine
- → Sucralose

What About the Keto Flu?

During the first few days on the keto diet, your body will quickly release its stored fluids. This is what accounts for losing water weight, but it can also lead to dehydration from a loss of electrolytes along with the water. Many people talk about experiencing a "keto flu" when trying a ketogenic diet for the first time; however, symptoms of "keto flu" are the same as clinical dehydration and can easily be avoided with these tips:

Stay hydrated! As a general rule, you should consume half of your body weight in ounces, so if you weigh 200 pounds, aim for 100 ounces of water a day. This can come in the form of unsweetened teas, seltzers, or lemon/lime-infused waters.

Keep up your electrolytes. The four main electrolytes are sodium, potassium, calcium, and magnesium. Avocados are high in potassium and magnesium. Nuts, seeds, and fatty fish such as salmon and mackerel are good sources of magnesium. You can also drink some chicken or beef broth, which is high in sodium, to boost electrolytes. However, if you are on a medically supervised low-sodium diet, consult with your doctor before increasing sodium levels.

Attack carb cravings with fat! You are trying to retrain your cells to look for fat as a primary fuel source rather than glucose from carbs. By giving those cells fat when a craving for sugars or carbs hits, you are reinforcing this process and encouraging your body to make the transition.

KETO FAQ

Do I need to restrict calories on keto?

Calories always matter in the end, especially if your goal is weight loss, but with keto, eating fewer calories occurs naturally. One of the most significant benefits of keto eating is appetite suppression. By eating greater amounts of fat and moderate amounts of protein, you stay satiated for longer, which allows you to eat fewer calories overall.

How much weight can I lose on keto, and how long will it take?

Weight loss is different for everyone. Much of your success will depend on how much weight you have to lose and how closely you follow the guidelines. That said, keto is known for stimulating rapid weight loss. A significant amount of water weight, 10 pounds or more, can be lost in the first few days or couple of weeks, and even more over the first month. After that, the loss continues but depends on your individual journey.

Do I need any special supplements for keto?

Electrolyte supplementation (sodium, potassium, magnesium) is essential on keto because you've restricted carbohydrates, which are responsible for water retention. You can make up for the loss by adding supplements, drinking more liquids with electrolytes (such as bone broth), and eating a variety of healthy whole foods. Exogenous ketones, MCT oil, and other supplements are not necessary for keto success, but they can be helpful.

Can I drink alcohol on keto?

The short answer is yes. Although sugary cocktails such as piña coladas and margaritas are out, an occasional low-carb beer or glass of white wine (reds are a little higher in carbs) is okay. Liquors such as vodka, whiskey, tequila, rum, and others are typically carb free (as long as they are not flavored—check labels) and are great with sugar-free mixers or over ice. Just be aware that the body burns through alcohol before anything else, so although it might not kick you out of ketosis, it could slow down weight loss. Also, with the lack of carbs in your body, alcohol affects you very quickly, so be cautious about how much you're drinking.

Do sugar alcohols kick you out of ketosis or slow weight loss?

Different sugar alcohols have varying effects on different people. Some people can eat prepackaged cookies, cakes, and other goodies and experience no issues, whereas others eat the smallest amounts and get kicked right out of ketosis. It's generally easier to stay in ketosis using sugar alcohols in homemade recipes instead of eating prepackaged treats—it's much less expensive, as well.

How long does it take to go full keto?

Once you get through the first week of the diet and past the keto flu (if one occurs), your appetite will be suppressed and you'll start feeling the benefits of ketosis. Within a couple of weeks, most people are much more familiar with what foods to eat and what to order in restaurants and are able to prepare a variety of keto-friendly meals and snacks. This book includes a 4-Week Meal Plan (page 35) to help you during the first month of your keto journey.

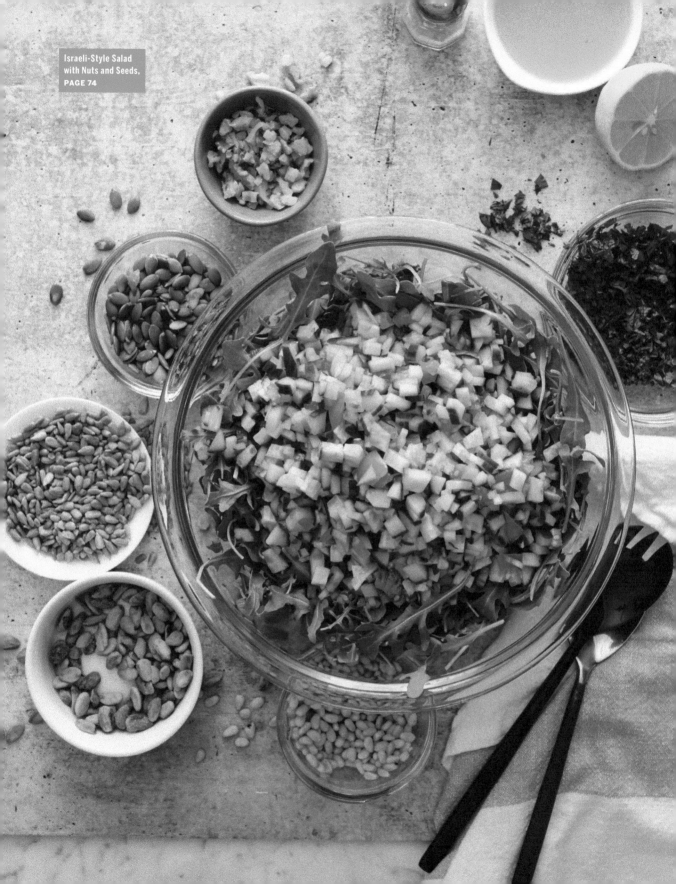

Israeli-Style Salad
with Nuts and Seeds,
PAGE 74

CHAPTER 2

Preparing for Success

Before you begin any major lifestyle changes, it's important to set yourself up for success. Getting rid of any foods that are not keto approved and stocking your pantry with only keto-friendly options will make this transition much easier. If you're not used to cooking at home, you may want to pick up a few kitchen gadgets, but almost every recipe can be adapted to the equipment you already have.

STOCKING YOUR KETO PANTRY

Many of the following ingredients will appear over and over in the recipes in this book. Keeping these pantry staples on hand will make preparing healthy meals at home easy and efficient. It's especially important to keep a number of keto-friendly condiments and spices on hand (or make them yourself; see chapter 12, page 179) to add flavor to the recipes.

Apple cider vinegar: Look for apple cider vinegar with "mother"—these are the probiotics that are fantastic for hunger suppression and overall gut health.

Avocado oil: If you use only one type of oil, avocado is the way to go. It shines in baking recipes as well as salad dressings and, because of its high smoke point, is perfect for searing.

Chicken broth: A staple for sauces and soups, chicken stock is an ingredient that should always be in your pantry. It's also great for sipping between meals to keep your electrolytes up.

Cocoa powder: This adds chocolate flavor to baking recipes, though on its own is very bitter. Use cocoa powder with keto-friendly sweeteners for making sugar-free baked goods.

Erythritol: One of the most common keto-friendly sweeteners, erythritol is used in both savory and sweet recipes. It doesn't spike glucose levels the way some other artificial sweeteners do.

Garlic: This is one of those ingredients that can go in just about any savory recipe. You can buy fresh bulbs of garlic, already peeled cloves, or jarred minced garlic for convenience.

Hot sauce: This is a must-have condiment for anyone who enjoys spicy foods. There are hundreds of types of hot sauce to choose from. Check the label and make sure there is no added sugar.

Mayonnaise: Most conventional brands of mayonnaise use low-quality oils, but there are a number of brands that use high-quality oil—look for those that use avocado or olive oil. You may also want to experiment with making your own Keto Mayonnaise (page 186).

Mustard: This pantry staple can be used for a variety of sauces or dressings and comes in a wide range of styles and flavors. Be sure to avoid mustard sweetened with honey or sugar.

Nuts: Walnuts and pecans are two low-carb, high-fat nuts that are a wonderful topping on salads as well a quick snack. Be careful with portions, however; it's easy to overeat because nuts are very calorie-dense.

Parmesan cheese: Because Parmesan is a hard, dry cheese, it's very low in lactose, making it easier to digest than other cheeses. It's a great addition to salads and is also used to thicken and flavor sauces.

Pickles: Whether whole, sliced, in spears, or in chips, pickles are a fantastic low-carb, low-calorie snack. Be sure to only buy pickles with no added sugar.

Pork rinds: One of the best ingredients for dips, pork rinds provide a salty, satisfying crunch to many keto recipes. Crushed pork rinds are also a bread crumb substitute.

Spice blends: Having a variety of spice blends helps keep your meals fresh and exciting. Buying blends also saves money because you don't have to buy as many individual spices.

New Keto Ingredients

On keto, you'll be avoiding grains and sugar, but there are a number of new and exciting alternative ingredients you can use to make low-carb versions of your favorite recipes.

Allulose: Used in both savory and sweet recipes, allulose is a low-carb, low-calorie sweetener with the taste and texture of real sugar but little to no impact on the body's glucose levels. Unlike erythritol, allulose doesn't have a cool aftertaste and has less impact on the gastrointestinal system.

Chia seeds: These little seeds become gel-like when soaked in liquid and can be used to thicken smoothies and shakes. They also make a nutrient-packed addition to grain-free granola and cereal.

Coconut aminos: A keto-friendly substitute for soy sauce, coconut aminos is made by extracting the sap from coconuts and turning it into a sweet and salty sauce. Coconut aminos is gluten-free and only has about 1 carb per teaspoon.

Hearts of palm noodles: This pasta substitute is made from a single ingredient and has a firmer texture than zucchini noodles. You can find hearts of palm noodles online or at health food shops. Hearts of palm noodles are gluten-free, low-carb, high-fiber, and one of the best pasta substitutes available.

MCT oil: Short for medium chain triglycerides, MCT oil is a fat source commonly used in shakes, smoothies, and Bulletproof Coffee (page 54) to add healthy fats to keto meals. Using a small amount of MCT oil in recipes can help suppress hunger and promote fat loss.

Sugar-free barbecue sauce: More and more brands, such as AlternaSweets and Sweet Baby Ray's, are making low-carb, sugar-free barbecue sauces. As always, check your labels to make sure there are no low-quality ingredients such as vegetable oil or MSG.

TOOLS AND EQUIPMENT

Aside from standard equipment such as pots and pans, wooden spoons, and mixing bowls, these are the kitchen tools that will help make your keto journey successful.

Dutch oven: A Dutch oven is a cast-iron pot with a lid and is used for making a variety of soups, stews, and sauces. Dutch ovens retain heat and are oven-safe, making them great for slow simmering and braising recipes. You can use a Dutch oven in place of a slow cooker.

Food processor: Look for a food processor with multiple attachments for shredding and dicing. Some even have a smaller, bullet-style attachment for making dressings and smoothies. Food processors are great for crushing pork rinds into bread crumbs as well as chopping meats and veggies for many of the recipes in this book.

Immersion blender: If you need to blend something quickly and don't want to make a mess, an immersion blender is a great option—just dip this stick blender right into the pot with your sauce and blend until smooth. Some immersion blenders have a whisk attachment that's very handy for making whipped cream.

Parchment paper sheets: This may seem unnecessary, but precut parchment paper sheets will save you hours of cleanup. The precut sheets are fitted for half-size sheet pans and will keep anything you're cooking from sticking. After you're done cooking, discard the parchment paper and rinse your pan clean in seconds.

Muffin pans: These are great for portion control and can be used for both sweet and savory recipes, such as Egg Breakfast Muffins (page 63) or Applesauce Yogurt Muffins (page 64). You can purchase traditional metal muffin tins or try the silicon variety—they make it very easy to remove the muffins from the flexible mold.

Waffle maker: You can prepare both sweet and savory recipes using a waffle maker. There are small, individual-portion models as well as larger ones that can make four waffles at a time.

SMART SHOPPING

Paying higher prices for grass-fed, free-range, organic foods buys you peace of mind on the ketogenic diet. These types of product are generally higher in good fatty acids and lower in not-so-great ones. If you're splurging on high-quality products, here's how you can cut costs elsewhere.

1. **Buy from a butcher or local farmer.** Butcher shops tend to be less expensive than most supermarkets, and you can also get excellent, less costly cuts such as the lesser known tri-tip. If you're cooking for the whole family or simply want lots of leftovers, make the slow cooker your friend and take advantage of roasts instead of single cuts of meat. If you have ample freezer space, consider buying a whole cow—seriously. Many farmers sell whole, half, or quarter cows and will butcher the meat and vacuum seal every cut for you.

2. **Shop every week.** When you come home to an empty refrigerator, it's hard to resist the urge to dine out or order in. But to do so while following a ketogenic diet usually means you're getting a cheap salad or an expensive steak, neither of which are fantastic options. A well-stocked refrigerator translates to nutritious meals for far less money than eating out.

3. **Create a meal plan.** On the ketogenic diet, you won't need most dried and packaged goods. Instead, you'll be buying a lot of fresh produce, meats, and dairy products that don't have a very long shelf life. Plan a week's worth of meals, along with a shopping list, and avoid veering from that list. By following a plan and a list, you'll avoid wasting food. Take advantage of the 4-Week Meal Plan (page 35) in this book where all the planning work is done for you.

4. **Shop the sales and cheaper cuts of meat.** You don't need to eat grass-fed, rib-eye steaks every day. If beef isn't on sale, look for less expensive options, such as chicken legs or pork chops. You can easily feed a family of four for under $5 if you buy meat on sale.

5. **Splurge on the essentials now.** Buy staples such as ghee, coconut oil, and dried herbs and spices in bulk from discount outlets. Your pantry will be well stocked, and your week-to-week grocery bill won't get blown up with tiny $15 jars of coconut oil at the grocery store. Most of these products have long shelf lives, and a little goes a long way, so it will be a while before you need to restock.

6. **Make your own.** Lots of recipes call for chicken broth. Next time you roast a chicken (or other type of roast), make your own Basic Broth, Chicken Variation (page 180). Strain the broth through cheese-cloth and freeze individual portions for future recipes. Instead of buying fresh herbs every week, make herbal ice cubes. Mince fresh herb(s) and pack them into ice cube trays so that each cube is about three-fourths full. Fill the trays with boiling water to blanch the herbs, then put them in the freezer. Pop the ice cubes out when they're frozen and store them in freezer bags.

7. **Invest in a vacuum sealer.** When you buy meat in bulk, make it last longer with a vacuum sealer. I even marinate my meats with spices and herbs (but not salt) before freezing.

8. **Focus on cheaper ingredients.** A whole-food approach to the ketogenic diet doesn't mean red meat every night. Tuna salad on romaine lettuce leaves, or slices of tomato and mozzarella drizzled with herbs, olive oil, and balsamic vinegar, is far more budget friendly and equally delicious.

9. **Buy in season.** Imported strawberries are expensive in December, but in the summer, you can get them at even the most expensive farm stand for under $3 a container. Buy in season and save on the fruits and vegetables that are abundant at different times of the year.

10. **Make recipes with fewer ingredients.** Herb garnishes make food look beautiful, but if they don't affect the flavor of the dish, you can eliminate them. You can cherry-pick the recipes you make based on the ingredients required. Ingredients that tend to increase the cost of a recipe include fresh herbs, fancy cheeses, and wine.

TIPS FOR SUCCESS

When you're first starting out on a ketogenic diet, there are lots of things to take into account and keep track of. The following tips will help you turn this way of eating into a lifestyle.

Meal Planning and Prep

Having a meal plan to follow, especially during the first month or two when you aren't sure what is or isn't keto friendly, can take the stress out of trying to decide what to cook every day. Following this book's 4-Week Meal Plan (page 35) for even a few weeks can get you off on the right foot and help create a rhythm that you'll be able to sustain long-term.

Helpful Tracking Tools

If you're not using a meal plan, it's incredibly important to track your meals and snacks to ensure you're meeting your macros. There are a number of helpful fitness trackers; my personal favorite is MyFitnessPal. You can enter specific foods you've eaten, or store recipes that you make often. If you're not technologically savvy, a good old-fashioned food journal works as well. As long as you are keeping track of everything you eat and drink throughout the day, you can stay on top of your macros.

Eating Out

Eating out can be a tricky endeavor when you first start following a ketogenic lifestyle, because you can't always be certain what's in your food. Your best bet is to do your homework on the restaurant ahead of time and plan what you are going to order. Many national chains have their nutritional information listed online so you can see if the ingredients are keto friendly. When in doubt, ask for sauces and dressing to be served on the side, and for sandwiches without the bun. There's also nothing wrong with ordering a steak with a side of broccoli and butter.

Cravings

No matter how strong your will or focus, cravings are inevitable. When a craving hits, first drink a big glass of water (a good idea to do throughout the day regardless). If you are still hungry, try doing 1 minute of exercise, such as running in place or doing arm circles. Getting the heart rate up can often dissipate hunger signals. If you are still having cravings, choose a snack high in protein and fat. Keep foods such as canned tuna and cooked chicken available at all times. Eat a few hundred calories and then wait 10 minutes. If you are still hungry, have a little more. The goal is to satisfy the craving but not overeat.

Supplements

Supplements are a source of controversy within the keto community. You should strive to get everything you need from food first, but if you find that you need to incorporate supplements such as electrolytes or magnesium, that's totally fine. I take vitamin D supplements daily to keep my immune system at its peak, but I also try to make sure I get as much sunlight as possible. However, keep in mind that if a supplement makes a claim that sounds too good to be true, it probably is. Supplements can help fill the gaps in your diet, but they shouldn't be the main source of your nutrition, and they aren't necessary for success. Always consult with your doctor before adding supplements to your diet.

EXERCISE

Outside of your diet, exercise is the most important factor in maintaining a healthy lifestyle. You don't need a fancy gym membership or expensive equipment to exercise. You just need to carve out a small amount of time each day to make sure you get active. Short walks and simple body weight exercises are a great place to start.

Contrary to popular belief, you don't need carbs to exercise or be active. Your body can burn ketones and fat as an energy source just as easily to help you gain muscle and lose fat. Try to make time each day for activity and gradually add a few more minutes than the previous day. Adding just five extra minutes of

Intermittent Fasting and Keto

In the past, dietitians have recommended three meals a day with up to three snacks between meals to increase your metabolism and prevent hunger. Recent research suggests that the opposite is healthier: eating less frequently, commonly called fasting.

Many people combine keto with intermittent fasting to get through a plateau in their efforts to lose weight. Once you obtain ketosis, fasting becomes easier, and the fat you burn comes from your own stores, not simply the extra fat you are eating.

The key to healthy fasting is making sure you are controlling *when* you eat, rather than just not eating at all. Many people confuse fasting with starving. Fasting is about manipulating *the timing* of your calorie intake. Some fasting plans call for calorie reduction, and it's important to ensure that you are getting enough nutrients, so if you are planning to fast, please do so responsibly.

There are a few methods of intermittent fasting, so you can audition one style at a time and see which works best for your lifestyle, though intermittent fasting is not required for keto.

The Leangains Approach (16/8 method): Fast for 16 hours and eat only within an 8-hour window, say 10 a.m. through 6 p.m.

The 5:2 Regimen: Eat only 500 to 600 calories for two days per week. During the rest of the week, eat your normal calorie allotment.

The Eat-Stop-Eat Plan: Fast for 24 hours, once or twice a week.

Alternate-Day Fasting: Fast for 24 hours, then eat your normal amount for the next 24 hours, then fast again, and so forth.

The Warrior Diet: Popularized by fitness expert Ori Hofmekler, this diet promotes eating very minimally during the day and then chowing down on a feast during a four-hour eating window.

activity per day can grow into consistent weight loss and added energy. Break your activity into three main categories: low-impact cardio, strength training, and high-impact cardio.

Low-Impact Cardio

Low-impact cardio is a great place to start if you're coming from a mostly sedentary lifestyle. Even a 15-minute walk after lunch or dinner will burn some calories and help you incorporate healthy habits into your daily routine. You may experience some soreness at first, but this is to be expected. The body is using muscles it hasn't used in a while, so it will take a little time to adapt. Start slowly and build up your routine—two or three workouts per week is a great beginning point.

Strength Training

Strength training is important for building and maintaining muscle. The more muscle you have, the more fat you will burn. The same rules apply to starting your strength training—begin with light weights and pay attention to your form to avoid injury. As you get more and more comfortable, build up the amount of weight and number of reps over time. This is a long-term lifestyle change, so it's important to make incremental gains over the long haul for sustainable progress.

High-Impact Cardio

High-impact cardio is great for getting the heart rate up and burning maximum calories over a short amount of time. You can burn more calories using short interval training such as HIIT, which stands for high-intensity interval training. A HIIT workout involves 30 seconds of high-intensity exercise followed by 90 seconds of rest or low-intensity exercise. Using resistance bands or light weights during a HIIT workout allows you to get a little strength training in at the same time. Start with at least 4 rounds of high-intensity exercises and work your way up to 8, 10, and 12 rounds. As you get stronger, you will find it easier to complete each circuit. Try the following exercises to get started.

QUICK HIIT ROUTINE

Do as many reps as you can in 1 minute for each of the following exercises (rest for 15 to 30 seconds between each exercise). Repeat the entire circuit 4 times.

One Minute of Jumping Jacks

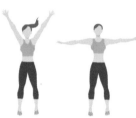
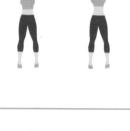

- → Start in a standing position with your feet together and your arms by your sides.
- → Jump your feet out to the side while simultaneously raising your hands over your head.
- → Immediately jump back to the starting position.
- → Repeat this sequence in a rhythmic motion.

One Minute of High Knees

- → Start in a standing position with your feet hip-distance apart and your arms by your sides.
- → Lift one knee toward your chest as high as possible while raising your opposite arm in a runner's position.
- → Return to the starting position and quickly lift the other knee and arm in the same manner.
- → Repeat this sequence in a fast motion.
- → **Advanced Option:** Jump as you lift each knee to your chest.

One Minute of Back Lunges (30 Seconds Each Leg)

- → Start in a standing position with your feet hip-distance apart and your hands on your hips.
- → With your right foot, take a large step backward, bending your knee at a 90-degree angle so your shin is parallel to the ground.
- → Push off your right foot to return to the starting position.
- → Repeat the movement with the same leg for 30 seconds; switch to the other leg and perform the exercise for an additional 30 seconds.

One Minute of Triceps Dips

→ Sit on the floor with your knees bent in front of you and
your feet flat on the ground.

→ Position your arms behind your back, with your palms on
the floor and your fingers pointing forward.

→ Slowly lift your hips toward the ceiling so your butt is
no longer touching the ground and you are in a tabletop
position.

→ While maintaining this position, gently bend your elbows
and then straighten them.

→ Repeat this bend and straighten movement for 20 seconds. Rest briefly,
and repeat 2 more times.

One Minute of Forearm Plank Hold

→ Lie facedown on the ground.

→ Lift yourself up to balance on your forearms (your forearms should be touching the ground) and your toes.

→ Make sure your hands are flat, your elbows are directly
under your shoulders, your back is straight, your
navel is pulled in, and your head is looking down at the
ground. Imagine creating a straight line from your shoulders to your feet.

→ Hold this position as long as you can, gently lower yourself to the ground,
and then repeat.

→ **Advanced Option:** Rather than balancing on your forearms, straighten
your arms while keeping your hands directly underneath your shoulders
to resemble a push-up position. Make sure to keep your back straight
and your core tight.

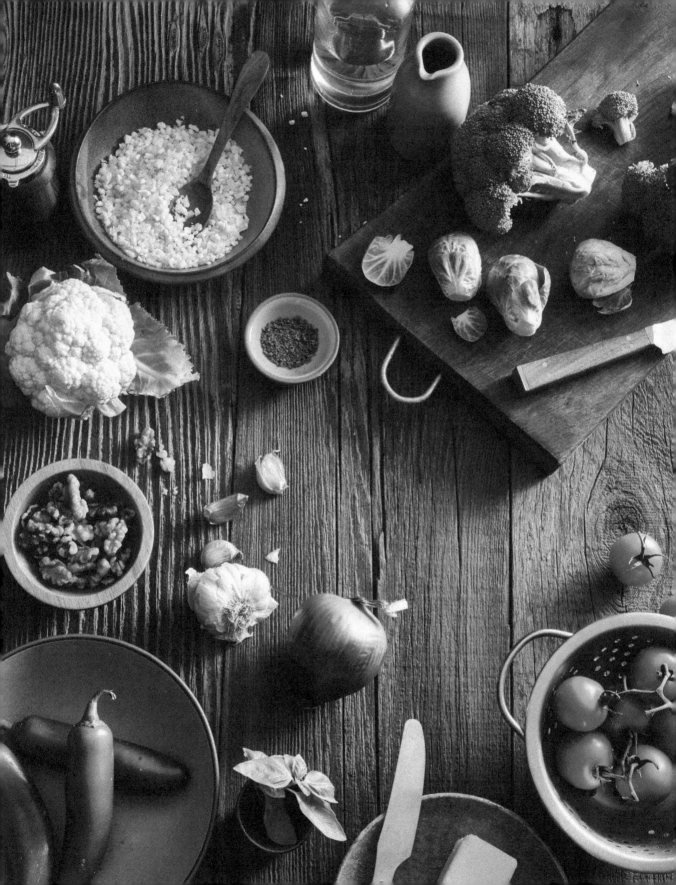

CHAPTER 3

Your Starter Meal Plans

To set yourself up for success, use this 4-week meal plan. Alongside easy, delicious recipes, you will find shopping lists and tips on the best ways to prep for the week, so you will always have meals ready to eat. Prepping ahead of time is very important and will help you stay on track and out of the snack drawer between meals.

ABOUT THE PLAN

Each week of this meal plan includes seven days of breakfast, lunch, and dinner. The breakfasts are all very simple to prepare or reheat, so you don't have to spend your mornings in the kitchen. Lunches will include salads as well as leftovers from previous dinners. To keep the meal plans cost-effective, you will reuse ingredients from recipe to recipe, but with lots of variation so you don't get bored. Do all your shopping at once and stick to the shopping list. If you only have healthy foods in your house, you won't be tempted by foods that can derail your success. The goal of this meal plan is to make the transition to a keto diet seamless, even if you have a busy lifestyle.

> **Note:** *One benefit of meal planning is using leftovers. These meal plans were designed for one person, so most recipes will yield leftovers. If a recipe in the meal plan only makes one serving, you'll see* 🥤 *next to it, which lets you know you should double the recipe when you prepare it so you can have leftovers later in the week. Portion out your dinners and store leftovers as soon as they are finished cooking so you're not tempted to overeat.*

A NOTE ON SNACKS

Snacks can be tricky—it's all too easy to overeat them. When you're craving a snack, ask yourself, "Am I hungry or am I bored?" Be honest with yourself. If you truly are hungry, keep a few savory snacks around, such as sugar-free jerky or pork rinds, as well as a few sweet snacks such as fresh berries or keto-friendly bars or cookies. High-fat, high-protein snacks will keep you satiated longer between meals. But be careful with nuts—they are very calorically dense. Always pre-portion nuts or buy 100-calorie snack packs to keep you on track.

WHAT TO EXPECT

When you first start the keto diet, you will probably feel hungry between meals. You are consuming fewer calories (and hopefully adding exercise to your routine), so your body will naturally want to eat more to compensate. During the first week, you may experience rapid weight loss—most of that is water weight. Use that initial weight loss to motivate you, knowing that every week won't be as dramatic. As you get into weeks 2, 3, and 4, you will start to feel less hungry due to the lack of sugar. This is where the body will really begin to convert into a fat-burning machine. By the end of the fourth week, you will be fully adapted and should find it much easier to adhere to the meal plans moving forward. If you feel lightheaded or experience any keto flu symptoms, make sure you are staying hydrated as well as consuming healthy fats and protein.

WEEK 1

Recipes in *italics* indicate leftovers from a previous meal.

DAY	BREAKFAST	LUNCH	DINNER
MONDAY	Chocolate Chia Pudding (page 58)	Chicken Salad–Stuffed Avocados (page 72)	Sirloin Steak with Creamy Mustard Sauce (page 141)
TUESDAY	*Chocolate Chia Pudding*	*Sirloin Steak with Creamy Mustard Sauce*	Caprese Balsamic Chicken (page 133)
WEDNESDAY	Mushroom Frittata (page 62)	*Chicken Salad–Stuffed Avocados*	*Caprese Balsamic Chicken*
THURSDAY	*Chocolate Chia Pudding*	Balsamic-Marinated Strawberry and Spinach Salad (page 70)	Bacon-Wrapped Scallops with Sweet Balsamic Sauce (page 112) and Cauliflower Mash (page 89)
FRIDAY	*Mushroom Frittata*	*Balsamic-Marinated Strawberry and Spinach Salad*	Turkey Taco Bowl (page 131)
SATURDAY	Keto Huevos Rancheros (page 61)	*Bacon-Wrapped Scallops with Sweet Balsamic Sauce and Cauliflower Mash*	*Turkey Taco Bowl*
SUNDAY	*Keto Huevos Rancheros*	Sirloin Steak with Creamy Mustard Sauce (page 141)	Crispy-Skin Salmon (page 111)

Shopping List

Protein

Bacon (1 pound)

Chicken breast, boneless skinless (2 pounds)

Salmon (12 ounces)

Sea scallops (6 ounces)

Sirloin steak (1 pound)

Turkey, ground, 93% lean (1 pound)

Dairy and Eggs

Butter (1 stick)

Cheese, cheddar (4 ounces)

Cheese, goat (4 ounces)

Cheese, mozzarella, shredded (4 ounces)

Cheese, Parmesan, grated (8 ounces)

Cream, heavy (whipping) (24 ounces)

Cream, sour (8 ounces)

Eggs (18)

Produce

Avocados (5)

Basil (1 bunch)

Cauliflower (1 head)

Cilantro (1 bunch)

Garlic (1 bulb)

Jalapeño (1)

Kale (5 ounces)

Lemons (2)

Lettuce, Boston (1 head)

Lettuce, romaine (2 heads)

Lime (1)

Mushrooms (8 ounces)

Onions, red (2)

Scallions (1 bunch)

Spinach, baby (4 ounces)

Strawberries (1 pint)

Tomato, medium (1)

Thyme (1 bunch)

Pantry

Apple cider vinegar

Chia seeds

Chili powder

Cinnamon, ground

Cocoa powder

Coconut aminos

Cumin, ground

Garlic powder

Italian seasoning

Mustard, Dijon

Mustard, grainy

Nutritional yeast

Oil, avocado

Oil, coconut

Oil, olive

Onion powder

Oregano, dried

Paprika, smoked

Pepper, black

Pepper, cayenne, ground

Pine nuts

Salsa

Salt

Vanilla extract

Vinegar, balsamic

Walnuts

WEEK 2

Recipes in *italics* indicate leftovers from a previous meal.

DAY	BREAKFAST	LUNCH	DINNER
MONDAY	Egg Breakfast Muffins (page 63)	½ recipe Tuna Melt (page 102)	Sloppy Joe Casserole (page 149)
TUESDAY	Blackberry Cheesecake Smoothie (page 56)	*Sloppy Joe Casserole*	Chicken Fajitas (page 129)
WEDNESDAY	*Egg Breakfast Muffins*	*Chicken Fajitas*	Pork Fried Rice (page 146)
THURSDAY	Lemon–Olive Oil Breakfast Cakes with Berry Syrup (page 67)	*Pork Fried Rice*	Cheeseburger Meat Loaf (page 140)
FRIDAY	*Lemon-Olive Oil Breakfast Cakes with Berry Syrup*	½ recipe Tuna Melt (page 102)	*Cheeseburger Meat Loaf*
SATURDAY	Blackberry Cheesecake Smoothie (page 56)	Barbecue Pork Bites (page 153) with Cauliflower Mac and "Cheese" (page 91)	Steak, Mushroom, and Pepper Kebabs (page 138)
SUNDAY	Easy Eggs Benedict (page 59)	*Steak, Mushroom, and Pepper Kebabs*	*Barbecue Pork Bites with Cauliflower Mac and "Cheese"*

Shopping List

Protein

Bacon (1 pound)

Bacon, Canadian
(8 slices)

Beef, ground 80% lean
(2 pounds)

Chicken thighs, boneless,
skinless (1 pound)

Pork tenderloin
(3 pounds)

Steak, sirloin (1 pound)

Tuna, 2 (5-ounce) cans

Dairy

Butter (2 sticks)

Cheese, cheddar,
shredded
(12 ounces)

Cheese, cheddar,
slices (4)

Cheese, cream, full-fat
(8 ounces)

Cream, heavy (whipping)
(16 ounces)

Cream, sour (½ cup)

Eggs (27)

Produce

Bell pepper, green (2)

Bell pepper, red (2)

Blackberries (4 ounces)

Cauliflower (3 heads)

Celery (2 stalks)

Cilantro (1 bunch)

Garlic (1 clove)

Ginger (2 ounces)

Lemons (4)

Lettuce, romaine
(1 head)

Mushrooms, white
button (8 ounces)

Onion, white (1)

Onion, yellow (1)

Parsley (1 bunch)

Scallions (1 bunch)

Spinach, baby
(8 ounces)

Frozen

Berries, mixed
(16 ounces)

Butternut squash, cubed
(12 ounces)

Pantry

Almond milk

Baking powder

Barbecue dry rub seasoning

Barbecue sauce, sugar-free

Celery seed

Chicken broth

Chives, dried

Cinnamon, ground

Coconut aminos

Coconut oil

Dill, dried

Erythritol

Flour, almond

Garlic powder

Ketchup, sugar-free

Mustard, Dijon

Mustard powder

Mustard, yellow

Nonstick cooking spray

Nutritional yeast

Oil, avocado

Oil, coconut

Oil, olive

Oil, toasted sesame

Onion powder

Paprika, smoked

Parsley, dried

Pepper, black

Red pepper flakes

Salt

Tahini

Tomato paste

Tortillas, low-carb (2 to 4)

Vanilla extract

Vanilla protein powder

Vinegar, white

Worcestershire sauce

WEEK 3

Recipes in *italics* indicate leftovers from a previous meal.

DAY	BREAKFAST	LUNCH	DINNER
MONDAY	Cacao Crunch Cereal (page 57)	Beef and Broccoli (page 145)	Mexican-Style Chicken Soup (page 75)
TUESDAY	Keto Huevos Rancheros (page 61)	*Mexican-Style Chicken Soup*	Casserole au Gratin (page 142)
WEDNESDAY	*Cacao Crunch Cereal*	*Casserole au Gratin*	*Beef and Broccoli*
THURSDAY	*Keto Huevos Rancheros*	Stuffed Bell Peppers (page 128)	Cubano Pork Chops (page 152)
FRIDAY	*Egg Breakfast Muffins (from week 2)*	*Cubano Pork Chops*	Steak and Egg Bibimbap (page 147)
SATURDAY	Lemon–Olive Oil Breakfast Cakes with Berry Syrup (page 67)	*Steak and Egg Bibimbap*	Crispy Fried Chicken Bites (page 118) with Pan-Roasted Green Beans (page 90)
SUNDAY	*Lemon–Olive Oil Breakfast Cakes with Berry Syrup*	*Crispy Fried Chicken Bites with Pan-Roasted Green Beans*	*Stuffed Bell Peppers*

Shopping List

Protein

Beef, ground, 80% lean (8 ounces)

Chicken breast, boneless skinless (1 pound)

Chicken thighs, boneless skinless (3)

Ham, sliced (1 pound)

Pork, ground (8 ounces)

Pork loin (2 pounds)

Steak, skirt (20 ounces)

Dairy and Eggs

Butter (1 stick)

Cheese, cheddar, shredded (8 ounces)

Cheese, mozzarella, shredded (½ cup)

Cheese, Parmesan, grated (8 ounces)

Cheese, Swiss, slices (4)

Cream cheese, full-fat (4 ounces)

Cream, sour (4 ounces)

Eggs, large (13)

Yogurt, whole milk, plain Greek (4 ounces)

Frozen

Beans, green (12 ounces)

Berries, mixed (12 ounces)

Cauliflower, riced (8 ounces)

Produce

Avocados (2)

Bell peppers, red (5)

Broccoli (2 heads)

Cauliflower, medium (2 heads)

Cilantro (1 bunch)

Cucumber (1)

Garlic (3 cloves)

Ginger, fresh (2 ounces)

Jalapeños (2)

Lemons (3)

Lettuce, Boston (1 head)

Lime (1)

Onion, white (1)

Onion, yellow (1)

Parsley (1 bunch)

Scallions (1 bunch)

Pantry

- Almonds, sliced
- Almonds, slivered
- Baking powder
- Basil, dried
- Chia seeds
- Chicken broth
- Cocoa nibs
- Coconut aminos
- Coconut, shredded, unsweetened
- Dill pickles, sliced
- Flour, almond
- Garlic powder
- Garlic salt
- Milk, nondairy
- Mustard, Dijon
- Mustard, yellow
- Oil, avocado
- Oil, coconut
- Oil, olive
- Onion powder
- Paprika, smoked
- Pepper, black
- Pork rinds
- Red pepper flakes
- Salsa
- Salt
- Sunflower seeds
- Taco seasoning
- Tomato sauce
- Tomatoes, diced
- Vanilla extract
- Vinegar, apple cider

WEEK 4

Recipes in *italics* indicate leftovers from a previous meal.

DAY	BREAKFAST	LUNCH	DINNER
MONDAY	Applesauce Yogurt Muffins (page 64)	Kale, Avocado, and Tahini Salad (page 73)	Avocado Chicken Burgers (page 127)
TUESDAY	Bulletproof Coffee (page 54)	Italian Sausage Soup (page 78)	*Kale, Avocado, and Tahini Salad*
WEDNESDAY	Kale and Chard Shakshuka (page 66)	*Avocado Chicken Burgers*	Black and Blue Chicken Thighs (page 123)
THURSDAY	*Applesauce Yogurt Muffins*	Zucchini Noodles with Avocado-Kale Pesto (page 98)	*Italian Sausage Soup*
FRIDAY	*Kale and Chard Shakshuka*	Shrimp à la Vodka Pasta (page 110)	*Black and Blue Chicken Thighs*
SATURDAY	*Egg Breakfast Muffins (from week 2)*	*Shrimp à la Vodka Pasta*	*Zucchini Noodles with Avocado-Kale Pesto*
SUNDAY	Belgian-Style Waffles (page 65)	Kale, Avocado, and Tahini Salad (page 73)	Crispy-Skin Salmon (page 111)

Shopping List

Meat and Seafood

Bacon, 2 slices

Chicken, ground
(1 pound)

Chicken thighs, boneless
skinless (1 pound)

Sausage, hot Italian
(8 ounces)

Shrimp, raw (1 pound)

Salmon (12 ounces)

Dairy and Eggs

Butter, unsalted (1 stick)

Cheese, blue crumbled
(4 ounces)

Cheese, Parmesan,
grated (8 ounces)

Cream cheese, full-fat
(4 ounces)

Cream, heavy (whipping)
(2 ounces)

Eggs (15)

Yogurt, whole milk, plain
Greek (4 ounces)

Produce

Avocados (4)

Basil (1 bunch)

Cucumber, seedless (1)

Garlic (2 bulbs)

Kale, chopped
(3 bunches)

Lemons (3)

Onion, white (1)

Parsley (1 bunch)

Scallions (1 bunch)

Spinach (5 ounces)

Swiss chard (2 bunches)

Tomatoes (2)

Zucchini (4 large)

Pantry

Almonds, slivered

Applesauce, unsweetened, 1 (4-ounce) container

Baking powder

Basil, dried

Black pepper, ground

Cajun seasoning

Cayenne pepper, ground

Chia seeds

Chicken broth (16 ounces)

Coconut aminos

Coffee, ground

Cinnamon, ground

Cumin, ground

Erythritol

Flaxseed meal

Flour, almond

Flour, coconut

Ginger, ground

Hearts of palm noodles

Low-carb buns (optional)

Marinara sauce, no-sugar-added

MCT oil powder

Nonstick cooking spray

Nutmeg, ground

Nutritional yeast

Oil, avocado

Oil, olive

Onion powder

Oregano, dried

Paprika, smoked

Pine nuts

Red pepper flakes

Salt

Stevia

Tahini

Tomatoes, canned, diced

Vanilla extract

Other

Vodka

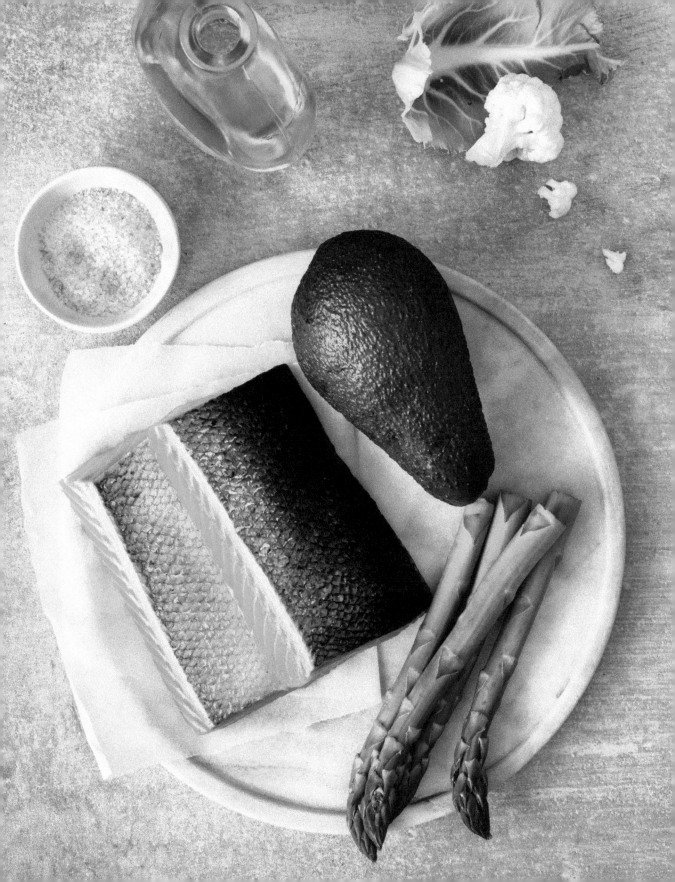

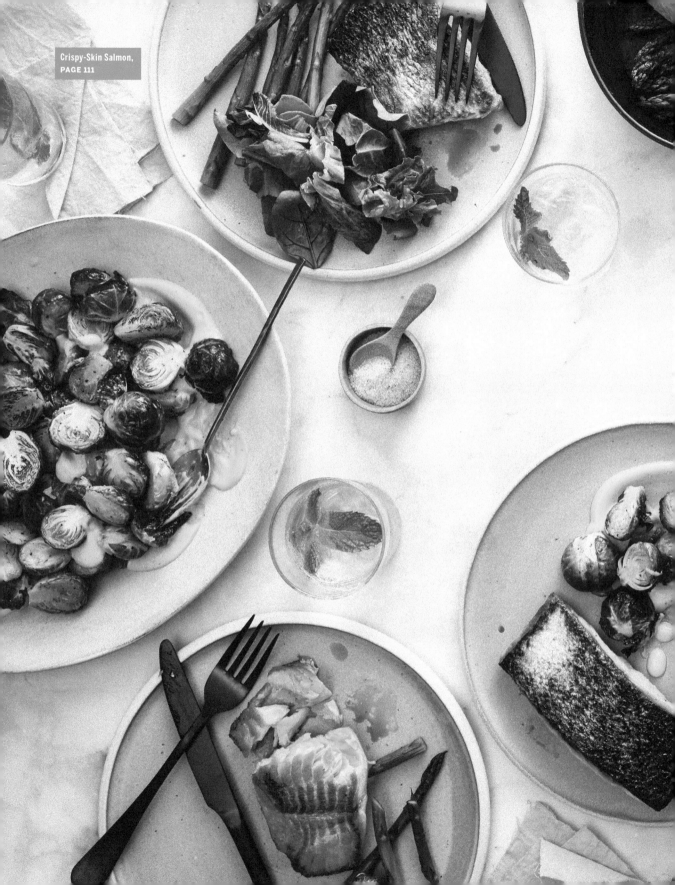

Crispy-Skin Salmon,
PAGE 111

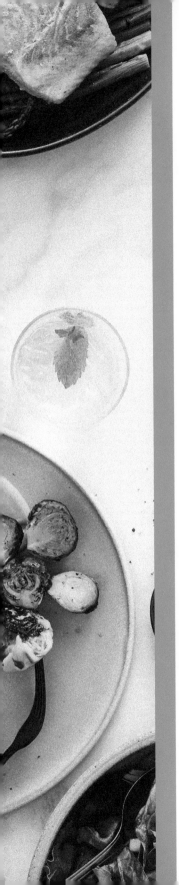

PART TWO

Easy Keto Recipes

The recipes in this book are made to yield from one to four servings, so if you're only cooking for yourself, you will have leftovers. On the other hand, if you're cooking for the whole family, you will probably want to double some of the recipes. No matter how many people you're feeding, doubling a recipe and freezing the leftovers is a great way to ensure that you'll always have food ready to go on nights when you might not be motivated to cook.

Each recipe has labels to let you know if a recipe can be prepared in 30 minutes or less, contains 5 ingredients or fewer (not including oil, salt, and pepper), or can be cooked entirely in one pot or pan. There are also tips for saving time, modifying recipes to fit different tastes, and how certain ingredients benefit your keto diet.

For those with other dietary restrictions, each recipe contains labels (gluten-free, nut-free, dairy-free, vegan, and vegetarian) to help you determine which recipes suit your needs. If you need to avoid gluten, always check the ingredient labels on packaged products to ensure the products were processed in a completely gluten-free facility.

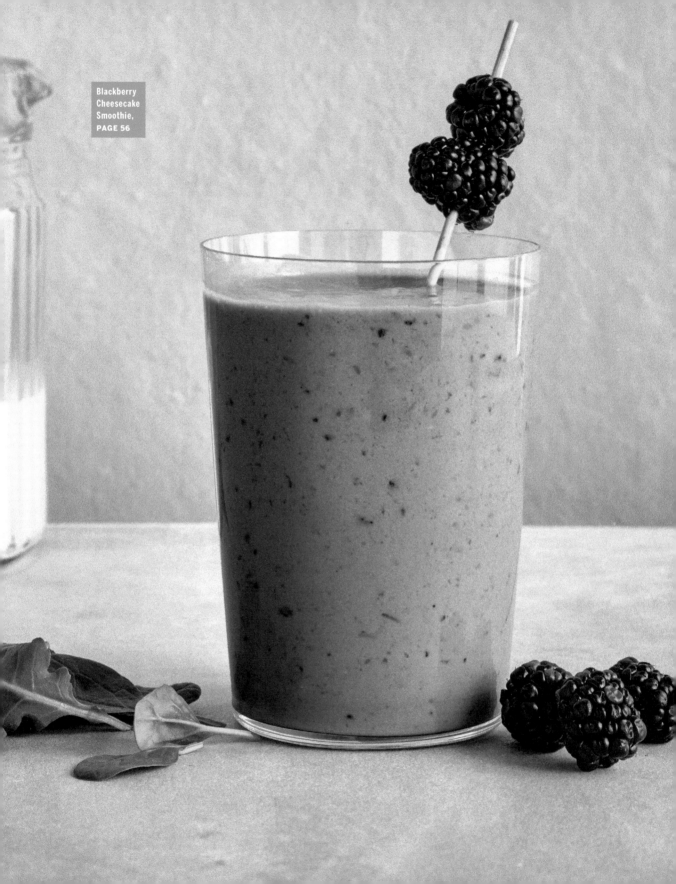

Blackberry
Cheesecake
Smoothie,
PAGE 56

Breakfast and Beverages

Bulletproof Coffee

5-INGREDIENT **30-MINUTE** **ONE POT** **GLUTEN-FREE** **NUT-FREE** **VEGETARIAN**

Bulletproof coffee is a staple beverage in many keto diets. The added fat plus the caffeine keeps you both full and energized long after you finish your cup.

SERVES 1
PREP TIME: 5 MINUTES

1½ cups hot coffee

2 tablespoons MCT oil powder or Bulletproof Brain Octane Oil

2 tablespoons butter or ghee

PER SERVING, REGULAR VERSION (ENTIRE RECIPE): Calories: 463; Total Fat: 51g; Protein: 1g; Total Carbs: 0g; Fiber: 0g; Net Carbs: 0g
MACROS: Fat: 99% / Carbs: 0% / Protein: 1%

PER SERVING, RAW EGG VARIATION (ENTIRE RECIPE): Calories: 270; Total Fat: 27g; Protein: 6g; Total Carbs: 0g; Fiber: 0g; Net Carbs: 0g
MACROS: Fat: 90% / Protein: 10% / Carbs: 0%

PER SERVING, PROTEIN AND COLLAGEN POWDER VARIATION (ENTIRE RECIPE): Calories: 476; Total Fat: 28g; Protein: 40g; Total Carbs: 17g; Fiber: 17g; Net Carbs: 0g
MACROS: Fat: 52% / Protein: 34% / Carbs: 14%

PER SERVING, SPICED VARIATION (ENTIRE RECIPE): Calories: 463; Total Fat: 51g; Protein: 1g; Total Carbs: 0g; Fiber: 0g; Net Carbs: 0g
MACROS: Fat: 99% / Protein: 1% / Carbs: 0%

1. Pour the hot coffee into a blender. Add the oil powder and butter. Blend until thoroughly mixed and frothy.

2. Pour into a large mug and enjoy.

RAW EGG VARIATION

To add protein, replace the MCT oil powder with 1 raw egg. It may sound strange, but the egg adds an appealing creamy texture, and although the hot coffee cooks the egg, there will be no hint of cooked proteins.

PROTEIN AND COLLAGEN POWDER VARIATION

You could also add a scoop or two of protein powder, such as Perfect Keto Collagen, which has a great chocolate flavor that is especially tasty in coffee. The collagen powder contains grass-fed collagen, MCT oil powder, and protein powder. Collagen is a good anti-inflammatory addition.

SPICED VARIATION

Add 1 teaspoon of ground cinnamon and a little keto-friendly sweetener to your bulletproof mixture for a delicious spiced version.

TIP: If you're new to the keto diet, you will want to start slowly with Bulletproof Brain Octane Oil. It is powerful, so work your way up to 2 tablespoons over the course of a few weeks.

Mean Green Smoothie

30-MINUTE | ONE POT | GLUTEN-FREE | NUT-FREE | VEGAN

Boasting three types of leafy greens, this smoothie is perfect for an early morning boost or midday snack. The kale, spinach, and Swiss chard provide nutrients such as iron, magnesium, calcium, and vitamin C—all of which are necessary for a healthy mind and body. Add herbs, for example parsley or cilantro, for an extra kick of flavor.

SERVES 2
PREP TIME: 10 MINUTES

1½ cups crushed ice, divided

1 cup kale, tightly packed and stemmed

½ cup spinach, stemmed

½ cup Swiss chard, stemmed

½ cup water

2 tablespoons coconut oil

2 tablespoons chia seeds

1. Put ¾ cup of ice in a blender. Add the kale, spinach, and Swiss chard. Blend to combine.

2. Add the remaining ¾ cup of ice, water, coconut oil, and chia seeds.

3. Blend for 1 minute or until smooth, then serve.

TIP: Save time by using prewashed frozen spinach, kale, and—if available—Swiss chard. If using frozen greens, reduce the ice by ¼ cup.

PER SERVING (½ RECIPE): Calories: 293; Total Fat: 23.3g; Protein: 7.7g; Total Carbs: 14.6g; Fiber: 11.2g; Net Carbs: 3.4g
MACROS: Fat: 69% / Protein: 11% / Carbs: 20%

Blackberry Cheesecake Smoothie

30-MINUTE | **ONE POT** | **GLUTEN-FREE** | **VEGETARIAN**

Though you should limit your berry consumption on the keto diet, blackberries are extremely rich in fiber (about five grams in two-thirds of a cup) as well as vitamins C and K. Blackberry seeds are also a good source of protein, omega-3 fatty acids, and fiber, so don't strain this smoothie after blending.

SERVES 2
PREP TIME: 10 MINUTES

1 cup unsweetened almond milk

3 ounces full-fat cream cheese

½ cup fresh or frozen blackberries

½ cup shredded baby spinach

1 scoop vanilla protein powder

1 tablespoon erythritol

1. In a blender, combine the almond milk, cream cheese, blackberries, spinach, protein powder, and erythritol and blend until smooth.

2. Pour into two glasses and serve immediately.

TIP: This is not an overly sweet smoothie. The blackberries add a certain tartness, so drinking a large amount won't be overwhelming. You could use this entire recipe as one serving and enjoy a quick 754-calorie meal.

PER SERVING (½ RECIPE): Calories: 377; Total Fat: 29g; Protein: 19g; Total Carbs: 10g; Fiber: 5g; Net Carbs: 5g
MACROS: Fat: 70% / Protein: 10% / Carbs: 20%

Cacao Crunch Cereal

30-MINUTE | **ONE BOWL** | **GLUTEN-FREE** | **VEGAN**

Craving cereal without all the sugar? This healthy combination will give you that crunch and sweetness alongside a good dose of fiber and healthy fats. Feel free to add erythritol or a couple of berries for natural sweetness. Strawberries and cacao nibs are a delicious combination!

SERVES 2
PREP TIME: 5 MINUTES

½ cup slivered almonds

2 tablespoons unsweetened shredded or flaked coconut

2 tablespoons chia seeds

2 tablespoons cacao nibs

2 tablespoons sunflower seeds

Unsweetened nondairy milk of choice, for serving

1. In a small bowl, combine the almonds, coconut, chia seeds, cacao nibs, and sunflower seeds. Divide between two bowls.

2. Pour in the nondairy milk and serve.

PER SERVING (½ RECIPE, CEREAL ONLY): Calories: 325; Total Fat: 27g; Protein: 10g; Total Carbs: 17g; Fiber: 12g; Net Carbs: 5g
MACROS: Fat: 70% / Protein: 11% / Carbs: 19%

Chocolate Chia Pudding

GLUTEN-FREE **NUT-FREE** **VEGETARIAN**

High in omega-3 fatty acids and fiber, chia seeds are a great addition to any ketogenic diet. When added to liquids, such as in smoothies or in this pudding, they create a gummy texture that acts much like gelatin. It's important to warm the cream prior to adding the cocoa powder, or it won't dissolve into the liquid and you'll be left with chalky clumps.

SERVES 4
PREP TIME: 10 MINUTES, PLUS 6 HOURS TO CHILL

2 cups heavy cream

¼ cup unsweetened cocoa powder

1 teaspoon almond or vanilla extract

½ to 1 teaspoon ground cinnamon

¼ teaspoon salt

½ cup chia seeds

1. In a small saucepan, heat the heavy cream over medium-low heat to just below a simmer. Remove from the heat and allow to cool slightly.

2. In a blender, combine the warmed cream, cocoa powder, almond extract, cinnamon, and salt, and blend until the cocoa is well incorporated.

3. Stir in the chia seeds and let sit for 15 minutes, until thickened.

4. Divide the mixture evenly among four ramekins or small glass bowls and refrigerate for at least 6 hours or until set. Serve chilled.

TIP: Try a berry version of this easy pudding by replacing the cocoa powder with pureed berries and omitting the cinnamon, or try a nutty version by adding ¼ cup of almond or hazelnut butter.

PER SERVING (¼ RECIPE): Calories: 561, Total Fat: 53g; Protein: 8g; Total Carbs: 19g; Fiber: 12g; Net Carbs: 7g
MACROS: Fat: 83% / Protein: 5% / Carbs: 12%

Easy Eggs Benedict

Buttery hollandaise sauce covering a perfectly runny egg that's nesting on a toasted English muffin; eggs Benedict is truly a treat for the taste buds. This keto version uses the simple 90-Second Bread (page 182) and a blender hollandaise sauce.

SERVES 4
PREP TIME: 15 MINUTES
COOK TIME: 20 MINUTES

8 slices Canadian bacon

4 batches 90-Second Bread (page 182)

1 tablespoon white vinegar

8 large eggs plus 3 large egg yolks, divided

1 tablespoon freshly squeezed lemon juice

1/8 teaspoon smoked paprika

10 tablespoons melted butter

1. Preheat the oven to 325°F. Line a baking sheet with parchment paper.

2. Arrange the bacon in an even layer on the baking sheet. Bake for 10 minutes, flip, and bake for another 10 minutes until evenly crisp. Remove from the oven and set aside.

3. While the bacon is baking, make the bread. When each piece is cool enough to handle, slice in half and toast.

4. Bring a large pot of water to a boil over high heat and then reduce the heat to low. Stir in the vinegar.

5. One at a time, crack the whole eggs into the water. Multiple eggs can cook together, but you want to crack them in individually so they don't combine. Cook for 3 minutes or until the whites are set. Remove the eggs from the water with a slotted spoon.

6. While the eggs cook, combine the egg yolks, lemon juice, and paprika in a blender and blend on high speed for about 30 seconds, until mixed.

CONTINUED >>

7. Reduce the blender speed to its lowest setting. Drizzle in the melted butter and continue to blend for another 30 seconds or until completely incorporated.

8. To serve, top each toast slice with 2 bacon slices, 2 eggs, and the hollandaise sauce.

> **TIP:** To make this recipe vegetarian, replace the bacon with 4 cups of spinach sautéed in 2 tablespoons of olive oil for 3 to 5 minutes.

PER SERVING (¼ RECIPE): Calories: 852; Total Fat: 75g; Protein: 40g; Total Carbs: 8g; Fiber: 2g; Net Carbs: 6g
MACROS: Fat: 77% / Protein: 19% / Carbs: 4%

Keto Huevos Rancheros

30-MINUTE | **ONE PAN** | **GLUTEN-FREE** | **NUT-FREE** | **VEGETARIAN**

Huevos rancheros, or "rancher's eggs," is a Mexican breakfast dish beloved by people far and wide. This variation of the spicy dish includes avocados, which are high in nutrients and the healthy monounsaturated fat oleic acid that helps fill you up.

SERVES 4
PREP TIME: 15 MINUTES
COOK TIME: 5 MINUTES

1 tablespoon extra-virgin olive oil

8 large eggs

½ jalapeño pepper, seeded and finely chopped

8 large Boston lettuce leaves

½ cup salsa

½ cup sour cream

1 cup shredded cheddar cheese

1 avocado, pitted, peeled, and diced

4 teaspoons chopped fresh cilantro

1. In a large skillet, heat the olive oil over medium-high heat.

2. Add the eggs and jalapeño and scramble until they form light and fluffy curds, about 4 minutes in total. Remove the skillet from the heat.

3. Arrange the lettuce leaves on a serving plate and evenly divide the eggs, salsa, sour cream, cheddar cheese, avocado, and cilantro among the leaves. Serve.

TIP: Chopped cooked chicken or cooked ground beef works well as a protein-packed topping for this filling breakfast.

PER SERVING (¼ RECIPE): Calories: 418; Total Fat: 34g; Protein: 22g; Total Carbs: 9g; Fiber: 4g; Net Carbs: 5g
MACROS: Fat: 71% / Protein: 21% / Carbs: 8%

Mushroom Frittata

ONE PAN **GLUTEN-FREE** **NUT-FREE**

Frittatas are delicious and simple to make. Any type of mushroom will work in this recipe. If you want to use portobello mushrooms, scoop out the black gills so your eggs don't turn an unsightly gray.

SERVES 4
PREP TIME: 10 MINUTES
COOK TIME: 25 MINUTES

4 teaspoons olive oil

⅔ cup sliced fresh mushrooms

⅔ cup shredded spinach

4 bacon slices, cooked
  and chopped

7 large eggs, beaten

⅓ cup crumbled goat cheese

Sea salt

Freshly ground black pepper

1. Preheat the oven to 350°F.

2. Place a large, ovenproof skillet over medium-high heat. Pour in the olive oil and heat.

3. Sauté the mushrooms until lightly browned, about 3 minutes.

4. Add the spinach and bacon and sauté until the greens are wilted, about 1 minute.

5. Add the eggs and cook, lifting the edges of the frittata with a spatula so uncooked egg flows underneath, for 3 to 4 minutes.

6. Sprinkle the top with the crumbled goat cheese and season lightly with salt and pepper.

7. Bake until set and lightly browned, 10 to 15 minutes.

8. Remove the frittata from the oven and let it stand for 5 minutes. Cut into 4 wedges and serve immediately.

TIP: Feta cheese also tastes lovely with the other ingredients in this dish. Feta is higher in fat and lower in protein than goat cheese, so keep that in mind when considering your keto macros.

PER SERVING (⅙ RECIPE): Calories: 316; Total Fat: 27g; Protein: 16g; Total Carbs: 1g; Fiber: 0g; Net Carbs: 1g
MACROS: Fat: 80% / Protein: 16% / Carbs: 4%

Egg Breakfast Muffins

30-MINUTE **GLUTEN-FREE** **NUT-FREE**

These cheesy muffins are actually quiches without the crust baked in a muffin pan. Serve them hot out of the oven or chilled, depending on your preference. They also freeze well, so whip up a double batch for easy meals all month.

SERVES 4
PREP TIME: 5 MINUTES
COOK TIME: 15 MINUTES

1 tablespoon butter, for greasing

6 large eggs

1 cup heavy (whipping) cream

½ cup shredded cheddar cheese, plus 2 tablespoons

5 bacon slices, cooked and chopped

½ teaspoon chopped fresh cilantro

Pinch salt

Pinch freshly ground black pepper

1. Preheat the oven to 350°F.

2. Lightly grease 8 cups of a muffin pan with the butter and set aside.

3. In a medium bowl, whisk the eggs, cream, ½ cup of cheddar, bacon, and cilantro. Season with salt and pepper.

4. Evenly pour the egg mixture into the muffin cups.

5. Bake the muffins until they are cooked through and lightly browned, about 15 minutes.

6. Remove the muffin pan from the oven and increase the oven heat to broil.

7. Sprinkle the remaining 2 tablespoons of cheddar onto the muffins, broil until the cheese is melted and bubbly, about 1 minute, and serve.

TIP: You will be using bacon regularly in a ketogenic lifestyle because it provides a good ratio of fat and protein. Cooked bacon will keep for at least 1 week in the refrigerator, so cook up an entire pack to save time when you need to add it to recipes.

PER SERVING (2 MUFFINS): Calories: 346; Total Fat: 31g; Protein: 15g; Total Carbs: 2g; Fiber: 0g; Net Carbs: 2g
MACROS: Fat: 79% / Protein: 19% / Carbs: 2%

Applesauce Yogurt Muffins

30-MINUTE **GLUTEN-FREE** **VEGETARIAN**

Muffins are a popular grab-and-go breakfast for anyone who is short on time. These beauties are low in calories and have the perfect combination of fat and protein to get you through the morning. You can replace the Greek yogurt with sour cream if you want to add a little more fat to your meal.

MAKES 12 MUFFINS
PREP TIME: 10 MINUTES
COOK TIME: 20 MINUTES

½ cup almond flour

2 tablespoons flaxseed meal

½ teaspoon baking powder

½ teaspoon granulated stevia

½ teaspoon ground cinnamon

½ teaspoon ground nutmeg

¼ teaspoon ground ginger

¼ teaspoon sea salt

3 large eggs

½ cup whole milk, plain
  Greek yogurt

½ cup unsweetened applesauce

3 tablespoons butter, melted

1 teaspoon vanilla extract

1. Preheat the oven to 350°F.

2. Line a 12-cup muffin pan with paper liners and set aside.

3. In a large bowl, stir together the almond flour, flaxseed meal, baking powder, stevia, cinnamon, nutmeg, ginger, and salt.

4. In a medium bowl, whisk together the eggs, yogurt, applesauce, butter, and vanilla.

5. Add the wet ingredients to the dry ingredients and stir to blend.

6. Spoon the muffin batter evenly into the muffin cups.

7. Bake for about 18 minutes or until the muffins are golden and a knife inserted into the center of one comes out clean.

8. Cool the muffins on wire racks until just warm and serve.

TIP: Flaxseed is popular with anyone looking to add protein and healthy omega-3 fatty acids to their diet, such as bodybuilders or professional athletes. Heating it in the oven will not reduce the omega-3 fatty acid (alpha-linolenic acid) in this powerhouse seed, so flaxseed is a wonderful addition to baked goods.

PER SERVING (1 MUFFIN): Calories: 65; Total Fat: 5g; Protein: 2g; Total Carbs: 3g; Fiber: 1g; Net Carbs: 2g
MACROS: Fat: 71% / Protein: 15% / Carbs: 14%

Belgian-Style Waffles

30-MINUTE | **GLUTEN-FREE** | **VEGETARIAN**

A waffle station is a sign of a great breakfast buffet. However, traditional waffles are loaded with gluten and sugar, two ingredients that can kick your body out of ketosis. Fear not: These waffles come together even faster than the frozen kind and will keep your body in prime fat-burning mode.

MAKES 4 WAFFLES
PREP TIME: 5 MINUTES
COOK TIME: 10 MINUTES

4 large eggs

4 ounces full-fat cream cheese, at room temperature

¼ cup almond flour

2 tablespoons erythritol

1 tablespoon coconut flour

1 tablespoon melted butter

1 teaspoon vanilla extract

½ teaspoon maple extract (optional)

½ tablespoon baking powder

Pinch sea salt

1 tablespoon unsweetened almond milk (optional)

Nonstick cooking spray or butter, for greasing

1. Heat a waffle iron.

2. In a blender, combine the eggs, cream cheese, almond flour, erythritol, coconut flour, butter, vanilla, maple extract (if using), baking powder, and salt and blend on high speed until completely combined. Add the almond milk (if using) for a thinner consistency and blend again until combined.

3. Spray the waffle iron with cooking spray.

4. Pour ¼ cup of batter onto the waffle iron and cook for 2 to 3 minutes or until browned and slightly crisped on both sides.

5. Remove the waffle. Repeat steps 3 and 4 to make 3 more waffles.

6. Serve with your favorite toppings. Refrigerate leftovers for up to 3 days or freeze for up to 1 month.

TIP: Get creative with flavor extracts and toppings, as long as you keep them low-carb and keto friendly. You may want to try banana extract and walnuts, apple extract and a pinch of cinnamon, or lemon extract with blueberries.

PER SERVING (1 WAFFLE): Calories: 237; Total Fat: 20g; Protein: 10g; Total Carbs: 11g; Fiber: 1g; Net Carbs: 10g
MACROS: Fat: 74% / Protein: 17% / Carbs: 9%

Kale and Chard Shakshuka

ONE PAN | GLUTEN-FREE | NUT-FREE | VEGETARIAN

Shakshuka is a classic Middle Eastern breakfast dish. It's made of inexpensive ingredients such as tomatoes, eggs, greens, herbs, and cheeses. Tomatoes are the base of most shakshukas, including this recipe. Tomatoes contain lycopene, a potent antioxidant that may support heart health. And get this: When you cook tomatoes, you actually increase the lycopene content!

SERVES 4
PREP TIME: 15 MINUTES
COOK TIME: 20 MINUTES

¼ cup extra-virgin olive oil

½ medium white onion, diced

1 tablespoon minced garlic

4 cups chopped kale, stemmed

4 cups chopped Swiss chard, stemmed

½ cup chopped fresh parsley

1 (15-ounce) can diced tomatoes with juices

Juice of 1 lemon

1 teaspoon ground cumin

½ teaspoon red pepper flakes

8 large eggs

1 cup shredded Parmesan cheese

1. In a large skillet, heat the olive oil over medium-high heat.

2. Sauté the onion and garlic until softened, about 3 minutes.

3. Stir in the kale, Swiss chard, and parsley and sauté until the greens are wilted, about 8 minutes.

4. Stir in the tomatoes and their juices, lemon juice, cumin, and red pepper flakes and bring the mixture to a simmer.

5. Using the back of a spoon, make 8 wells in the tomato mixture, then crack an egg into each well. Cover the skillet with a lid and let cook until the egg whites are no longer translucent, 4 to 5 minutes.

6. Remove from the heat and serve topped with the Parmesan cheese.

TIP: This recipe can be prepared as individual portions in 6-ounce ramekins. Make the recipe up to step 4 and evenly divide the tomato mixture among four ramekins. Then, crack the eggs on top. Cover each ramekin and store in the refrigerator for up to two days. Bake straight from the refrigerator in a 375°F oven for about 30 minutes or until the eggs are cooked through and the tomato base is hot.

PER SERVING (¼ RECIPE): Calories: 407; Total Fat: 30g; Protein: 24g; Total Carbs: 13g; Fiber: 4g; Net Carbs: 9g
MACROS: Fat: 65% / Protein: 23% / Carbs: 12%

Lemon–Olive Oil Breakfast Cakes with Berry Syrup

30-MINUTE **DAIRY-FREE** **GLUTEN-FREE** **VEGETARIAN**

Weekends are made for pancakes! The lemon flavor in these breakfast cakes is a light and refreshing twist on a breakfast favorite.

SERVES 4
PREP TIME: 5 MINUTES
COOK TIME: 10 MINUTES

FOR THE PANCAKES

1 cup almond flour

1 teaspoon baking powder

¼ teaspoon salt

6 tablespoons extra-virgin olive oil, divided

2 large eggs

Zest and juice of 1 lemon

½ teaspoon vanilla or almond extract

FOR THE BERRY SYRUP

1 cup frozen mixed berries

1 tablespoon water or freshly squeezed lemon juice, plus more if needed

½ teaspoon vanilla extract

PER SERVING (2 PANCAKES WITH ¼ CUP BERRY SYRUP): Calories: 275; Total Fat: 26g; Protein: 4g; Total Carbs: 8g; Fiber: 2g; Net Carbs: 6g **MACROS:** Fat: 83% / Protein: 6% / Carbs: 11%

1. **To make the pancakes:** In a large bowl, combine the almond flour, baking powder, and salt, and whisk to break up any clumps.

2. Add 4 tablespoons of olive oil, the eggs, lemon zest and juice, and vanilla, then whisk well to combine.

3. In a large skillet, heat 1 tablespoon of olive oil. Spoon in about 2 tablespoons of batter per pancake, to make 4 pancakes at a time. Cook until bubbles begin to form, 4 to 5 minutes, then flip. Cook another 2 to 3 minutes on the second side. Repeat with the remaining 1 tablespoon of olive oil and remaining batter.

4. **To make the berry syrup:** In a small saucepan, heat the frozen berries, water, and vanilla for 3 to 4 minutes over medium-high heat, until bubbly, adding more water if the mixture is too thick. Using the back of a spoon or fork, mash the berries and whisk until smooth.

5. Divide the pancakes among four plates, drizzle with the syrup, and serve hot.

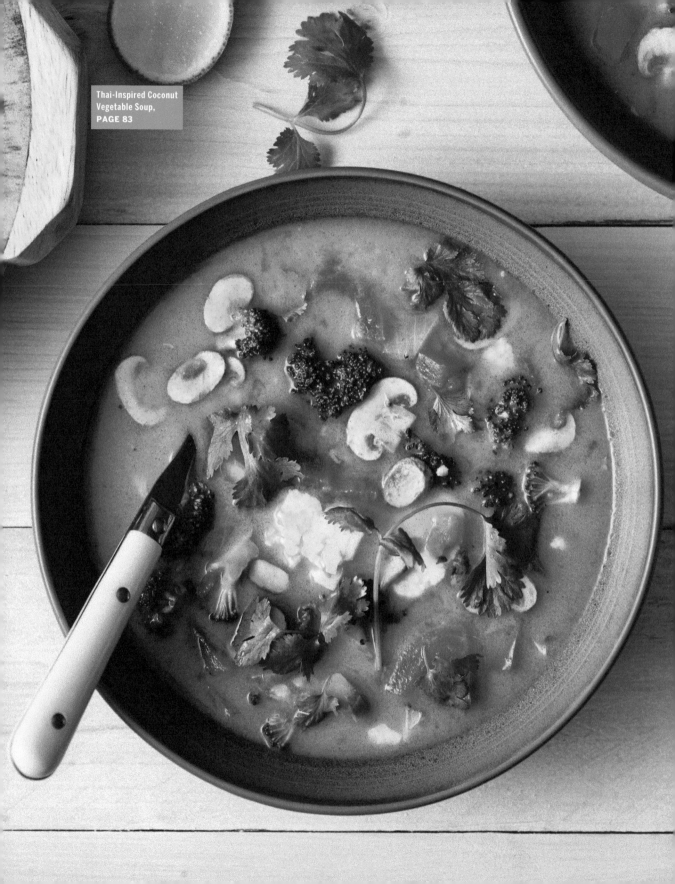

Thai-Inspired Coconut Vegetable Soup,
PAGE 83

CHAPTER 5

Soups and Salads

Balsamic-Marinated Strawberry and Spinach Salad

GLUTEN-FREE **VEGETARIAN**

Balsamic marinated strawberries are a fantastic balance of tangy and sweet—perfect when combined with the crunch of chopped walnuts and creamy crumbled goat cheese. The dressing is incredibly simple and uses the balsamic vinegar and olive oil that the strawberries are marinated in.

SERVES 1
PREP TIME: 15 MINUTES, PLUS 30 MINUTES TO MARINATE

¼ cup sliced strawberries

2 tablespoons balsamic vinegar

1 tablespoon extra-virgin olive oil

¼ teaspoon Italian seasoning

1 cup baby spinach

2 tablespoons crumbled goat cheese

2 tablespoons chopped walnuts

½ cup sliced red onion, or to taste

1 teaspoon Dijon mustard

1. Put the strawberries in a sealable container along with the balsamic vinegar, olive oil, and Italian seasoning. Cover and marinate in the refrigerator for 30 minutes.

2. In a salad bowl, layer the spinach, cheese, walnuts, and onion. Top with the marinated strawberries, reserving the marinade.

3. To the marinade, add the mustard and whisk vigorously until fully emulsified. You may also use a blender for this step.

4. Pour the dressing over the salad and serve.

TIP: The strawberries can be marinated for up to 24 hours ahead of time. You can also marinate the strawberries in a blender bottle used for protein shakes. Once you remove the strawberries, add the Dijon mustard and shake to combine.

PER SERVING (ENTIRE RECIPE): Calories: 327; Total Fat: 26g; Protein: 7g; Total Carbs: 17g; Fiber: 4g; Net Carbs: 13g
MACROS: Fat: 71% / Protein: 8% / Carbs: 21%

Chicken and Bacon Salad with Sun-Dried Tomato Dressing

30-MINUTE **DAIRY-FREE** **GLUTEN-FREE** **NUT-FREE**

If you don't want to make the dressing for this salad but still want the sun-dried tomato taste, you can use sun-dried tomatoes in place of the cherry tomatoes and drizzle the olive oil from the tomatoes over the top of the salad. Make sure any store-bought cooked chicken used for this salad doesn't contain any added sugar.

SERVES 1
PREP TIME: 10 MINUTES
COOK TIME: 5 MINUTES

2 slices bacon

3 sun-dried tomatoes (packed in olive oil)

1 tablespoon extra-virgin olive oil

1 teaspoon minced shallots

1 teaspoon nutritional yeast or grated cheese (optional)

½ teaspoon dried oregano

½ teaspoon freshly squeezed lemon juice (optional)

¼ teaspoon garlic powder

Pinch salt

Pinch freshly ground black pepper

1 cup Bibb or butter lettuce leaves

4 ounces cooked chicken breast and/or thigh meat, diced

¼ cup cherry tomatoes, halved

½ avocado, pitted, peeled, and diced

1. Heat a shallow skillet over medium heat. When warm, cook the bacon to your desired crispness, about 5 minutes. Turn off the heat and let the bacon sit in the skillet.

2. In a blender, combine the sun-dried tomatoes, olive oil, shallots, nutritional yeast (if using), oregano, lemon juice (if using), garlic powder, salt, and pepper. Blend until smooth.

3. Arrange the lettuce on a plate. Top with the chicken, cherry tomatoes, and avocado. Lay the bacon on top (alternatively, you can chop the bacon and sprinkle it on after you've dressed the salad). If you'd like, pour the bacon pan drippings over the salad (trust me, it's amazing).

4. Spoon on 1 to 2 tablespoons of dressing and dig in!

PER SERVING (ENTIRE RECIPE): Calories: 858; Total Fat: 62g; Protein: 52g; Total Carbs: 23g; Fiber: 14g; Net Carbs: 9g
MACROS: Fat: 65% / Protein: 24% / Carbs: 11%

Chicken Salad–
Stuffed Avocados

30-MINUTE | **ONE BOWL** | **GLUTEN-FREE** | **NUT-FREE**

Avocados make a handy, attractive container for this tasty chicken salad filling. If the hollow of the avocado is too shallow after you remove the pit, carefully scoop out a couple spoonfuls of green flesh to create more room. Either mash the removed avocado into the chicken salad or save it for another recipe.

SERVES 4
PREP TIME: 25 MINUTES

1½ cups chopped, cooked chicken

¼ cup Keto Mayonnaise (page 186) or store-bought mayonnaise

1 tablespoon chopped scallion, white and green parts

1 tablespoon freshly squeezed lemon juice

½ teaspoon smoked paprika

¼ teaspoon garlic powder

¼ teaspoon ground cayenne pepper

2 small avocados, halved and pitted

2 tablespoons grated Parmesan cheese

1. In a medium bowl, stir together the chicken, mayonnaise, scallion, lemon juice, paprika, garlic powder, and cayenne until well mixed.

2. Divide the chicken mixture evenly between the avocado halves, sprinkle each with Parmesan cheese, and serve.

TIP: Half an avocado with chicken salad is a hearty snack, but if you'd like to have this for a midday meal, portion a whole avocado per person and double the nutrition values.

PER SERVING (¼ RECIPE): Calories: 348; Total Fat: 28g; Protein: 17g; Total Carbs: 10g; Fiber: 7g; Net Carbs: 3g
MACROS: Fat: 69% / Protein: 21% / Carbs: 10%

Kale, Avocado, and Tahini Salad

30-MINUTE **ONE BOWL** **GLUTEN-FREE** **VEGAN**

Not only does this salad satisfy on so many fronts—hello, creamy and crunchy—it's also astoundingly detoxifying. Choose this salad when you are feeling a little run down and in need of a boost.

SERVES 4
PREP TIME: 5 MINUTES

1 bunch kale, stemmed, leaves
  cut into ribbons

¼ cup extra-virgin olive oil

4 to 5 tablespoons Tahini
  Goddess Dressing (page 189)

1 avocado, pitted, peeled,
  and sliced

¼ cup slivered almonds

3 tablespoons chia seeds

1. In a large mixing bowl, coat the kale with the olive oil. Massage the leaves with your hands to tenderize them and remove bitterness.

2. Toss the massaged kale with the dressing.

3. Divide the salad among 4 bowls and top each bowl with the avocado, almonds, and chia seeds.

TIP: This salad does well as a make-ahead item, so double the recipe and store half in an airtight container in the refrigerator. The kale will keep its texture for up to 3 days.

PER SERVING (¼ RECIPE): Calories: 370; Total Fat: 30g; Protein: 9g; Carbs: 22g; Fiber: 12g; Net Carbs: 10g
MACROS: Fat: 70% / Protein: 7% / Carbs: 23%

Israeli-Style Salad with Nuts and Seeds

30-MINUTE | **GLUTEN-FREE** | **VEGAN**

The most well-known national dish of Israel, according to some, this salad is a standard accompaniment to many Israeli meals. This beautifully simple version becomes a meal in itself with protein and healthy fats from a variety of nuts and seeds, which also gives it great texture and crunch.

SERVES 4
PREP TIME: 15 MINUTES
COOK TIME: 5 MINUTES

¼ cup pine nuts

¼ cup shelled pistachios

¼ cup coarsely chopped walnuts

¼ cup shelled pumpkin seeds

¼ cup shelled sunflower seeds

2 large English cucumbers, finely chopped

1 pint cherry tomatoes, finely chopped

½ small red onion, finely chopped

½ cup finely chopped fresh flat-leaf Italian parsley

¼ cup extra-virgin olive oil

2 to 3 tablespoons freshly squeezed lemon juice (from 1 lemon)

1 teaspoon salt

¼ teaspoon freshly ground black pepper

4 cups baby arugula

1. In a large dry skillet, toast the pine nuts, pistachios, walnuts, pumpkin seeds, and sunflower seeds over medium-low heat until golden and fragrant, 5 to 6 minutes, being careful not to burn them. Remove from the heat and set aside.

2. In a large bowl, combine the cucumbers, tomatoes, red onion, and parsley.

3. In a small bowl, whisk the olive oil, lemon juice, salt, and pepper. Pour over the chopped vegetables and toss to coat.

4. Add the toasted nuts and seeds and arugula and toss with the salad to blend well. Serve at room temperature or chilled.

PER SERVING (¼ RECIPE): Calories: 414; Total Fat: 34g; Protein: 10g; Total Carbs: 17g; Fiber: 6g; Net Carbs: 11g
MACROS: Fat: 74% / Protein: 10% / Carbs: 16%

Mexican-Style Chicken Soup

ONE POT **DAIRY-FREE** **GLUTEN-FREE**

You won't be able to get enough of this soup—a take on chicken tortilla soup, without the tortillas. I recommend making a triple batch so you can eat it all week long. It's even better topped with freshly diced avocado or a dollop of sour cream.

SERVES 2
PREP TIME: 10 MINUTES
COOK TIME: 30 MINUTES

2 tablespoons avocado oil

¼ medium white onion, diced

¼ red bell pepper, diced

1 garlic clove, minced

½ cup diced tomatoes, fresh or canned

1 tablespoon Taco Seasoning (page 183)

4 cups Basic Broth, Chicken Variation (page 180) or store-bought chicken broth

1 tablespoon minced fresh cilantro, plus more for garnish

3 cooked, boneless chicken thighs, shredded with a fork

Juice of ½ lime, plus more for serving

½ avocado, pitted, peeled, and diced

1. In a medium pot, heat the oil over medium heat until shimmering.

2. Add the onion, bell pepper, and garlic, and sauté for 5 to 7 minutes until soft.

3. Add the tomatoes and taco seasoning; stir well. Cook for 2 to 3 minutes until fragrant.

4. Add the chicken broth and cilantro and stir everything together.

5. Bring the soup to a boil, then reduce the heat to low and let it simmer for 20 minutes.

6. Add the cooked chicken and lime juice to the pot and stir together until everything is combined.

7. Garnish with the diced avocado, more lime juice, and extra cilantro.

PER SERVING (2 CUPS): Calories: 529; Total Fat: 41g; Protein: 31g; Total Carbs: 9g; Fiber: 4g; Net Carbs: 5g
MACROS: Fat: 70% / Protein: 23% / Carbs: 7%

Turkey Jalapeño Soup

ONE POT **DAIRY-FREE** **GLUTEN-FREE** **NUT-FREE**

If you enjoy simple, hearty soups, this recipe is for you. The jalapeño pepper adds a kick, plus there are onions, carrots, and cabbage for bulk, fiber, and flavor. All that fiber, by the way, helps fill you up. Make sure you follow the directions carefully and add the cabbage at the end. If cabbage simmers too long, it becomes slimy and smelly.

SERVES 4
PREP TIME: 15 MINUTES
COOK TIME: 20 MINUTES

3 tablespoons coconut oil

1 medium white onion, chopped

1 jalapeño pepper, seeded and chopped

1 tablespoon minced garlic

1 tablespoon peeled, grated fresh ginger

6 cups Basic Broth, Chicken Variation (page 180) or store-bought chicken broth

12 ounces cooked, diced turkey

2 cups full-fat canned coconut milk

1 carrot, diced

Zest and juice of 1 lime

1 cup shredded cabbage

2 tablespoons chopped fresh cilantro, for garnish

1. In a large stockpot, heat the coconut oil over medium-high heat until shimmering.

2. Add the onion, jalapeño, garlic, and ginger and sauté for about 5 minutes until softened.

3. Add the chicken broth, turkey, coconut milk, carrot, and lime zest and juice to the stockpot.

4. Bring the soup to a boil, then reduce the heat to low and simmer until the vegetables are tender, about 10 minutes.

5. Add the cabbage and simmer for 5 minutes until wilted.

6. Serve topped with the cilantro.

TIP: This soup can be doubled and frozen with no loss of taste or texture. Portion the soup into single servings in containers or freezer bags and thaw when ready to eat.

PER SERVING (¼ RECIPE): Calories: 482; Total Fat: 38g; Protein: 28g; Total Carbs: 12g; Fiber: 2g; Net Carbs: 10g
MACROS: Fat: 67% / Protein: 24% / Carbs: 9%

Slow Cooker Keto Chili

DAIRY-FREE **GLUTEN-FREE** **NUT-FREE**

This chili is great as either an intimate meal for two or a crowd-pleaser on game day. Be sure to adjust the recipe based on how many people you are feeding. This comes together in a slow cooker, so you can make it in advance and keep it warm until you're ready to serve it. Try creating a toppings bar with cheddar cheese, pickled jalapeños, diced onion, and sour cream.

SERVES 2
PREP TIME: 10 MINUTES
COOK TIME: 2 HOURS,
15 MINUTES

1 tablespoon avocado oil

¼ medium white onion, diced

¼ green bell pepper, diced

2 garlic cloves, minced

12 ounces 80% lean ground beef

2 cups Basic Broth, Beef Variation (page 180) or store-bought beef broth

1 (12-ounce) can tomato sauce

1 tablespoon coconut aminos

½ teaspoon ground cumin

½ teaspoon garlic powder

¼ teaspoon chili powder

¼ teaspoon smoked paprika

¼ teaspoon dried oregano

¼ teaspoon ground cayenne pepper

¼ teaspoon freshly ground black pepper

¼ teaspoon salt

1. In a large skillet, heat the oil over medium heat until shimmering.

2. Add the onion, bell pepper, and garlic and sauté for 5 to 7 minutes, until soft.

3. Add the ground beef and cook for about 5 minutes, until it is browned and no longer pink.

4. Drain any excess grease and transfer the mixture to a slow cooker.

5. Add the beef broth, tomato sauce, coconut aminos, cumin, garlic powder, chili powder, paprika, oregano, cayenne, black pepper, and salt. Stir to combine everything.

6. Cook on high for 2 hours, stirring occasionally, until the flavors have melded. Serve with your toppings of choice.

PER SERVING (2 CUPS): Calories: 586; Total Fat: 42g; Protein: 33g; Total Carbs: 21g; Fiber: 5g; Net Carbs: 16g
MACROS: Fat: 64% / Protein: 23% / Carbs: 13%

Italian Sausage Soup

30-MINUTE **ONE PAN** **GLUTEN-FREE** **NUT-FREE**

Soup is wonderful, especially in the fall and winter. This recipe makes a slightly spicy, comforting Italian sausage soup. With a nice big salad on the side, it's the perfect cold weather meal.

SERVES 4
PREP TIME: 5 MINUTES
COOK TIME: 25 MINUTES

1 tablespoon olive oil

½ medium white onion, diced

3 garlic cloves, minced

8 ounces hot Italian sausage, casings removed

2 cups Basic Broth, Chicken Variation (page 180) or store-bought chicken broth

1 (14.5-ounce) can diced tomatoes

1 to 2 teaspoons red pepper flakes

1 teaspoon dried oregano

1 teaspoon dried basil

Salt

Freshly ground black pepper

¼ cup freshly grated Parmesan cheese, divided

2 cups chopped spinach

1. In a large saucepan, heat the olive oil over medium heat until shimmering.

2. Add the onion and garlic. Sauté for 5 to 7 minutes until the onion is softened and translucent.

3. Add the sausage to the pan. Crumble and cook for about 5 minutes, allowing the meat to brown.

4. Stir in the chicken broth and tomatoes with their juices. Bring to a boil and reduce the heat to low.

5. Add the red pepper flakes, oregano, and basil. Season with salt and pepper and stir in 2 tablespoons of Parmesan.

6. Simmer for 10 minutes, until the flavors have melded. Remove from the heat.

7. Stir in the spinach until wilted. Serve sprinkled with the remaining 2 tablespoons of Parmesan.

KALE VARIATION

Use kale instead of spinach—add it to the pan with the onion and garlic. Follow the rest of the recipe as written.

CABBAGE VARIATION

Add ½ head of cabbage, sliced, to the pan with the onion and garlic. You can do this with the original recipe or as part of the kale variation (cabbage and kale are delicious together).

PER SERVING (¼ RECIPE): Calories: 365; Total Fat: 20g; Protein: 33g; Total Carbs: 11g; Fiber: 2g; Net Carbs: 9g
MACROS: Fat: 52% / Protein: 36% / Carbs: 12%

KALE VARIATION PER SERVING (¼ RECIPE): Calories: 377; Total Fat: 21g; Protein: 34g;
Total Carbs: 14g; Fiber: 2g; Net Carbs: 12g;
MACROS: Fat: 50% / Protein: 36% / Carbs: 14%

CABBAGE VARIATION PER SERVING (¼ RECIPE): Calories: 397; Total Fat: 21g; Protein: 35g;
Total Carbs: 17g; Fiber: 4g; Net Carbs: 13g
MACROS: Fat: 49% / Protein: 35% / Carbs: 16%

Seafood Chowder

ONE POT **GLUTEN-FREE** **NUT-FREE**

Chowder is historically a peasant food prepared in a large pot or *chaudière*, which is the French word for "cauldron." The ingredients of chowder include vegetables and often fish or seafood, depending on the area of the world. You can make this dish with mussels, different types of fish, scallops, or squid.

SERVES 4
PREP TIME: 20 MINUTES
COOK TIME: 25 MINUTES

4 tablespoons coconut oil

1 medium sweet onion, finely chopped

2 celery stalks, finely chopped

2 garlic cloves, minced

2 teaspoons xanthan gum

3 cups Basic Broth, Chicken Variation (page 180) or store-bought chicken broth

2 cups chopped cooked lobster meat

4 ounces cooked shrimp, chopped

1½ cups heavy (whipping) cream

1 teaspoon chopped fresh thyme

Sea salt

Freshly ground black pepper

2 tablespoons chopped fresh chives, for serving

1. In a large saucepan, melt the coconut oil over medium-high heat.

2. Add the onion, celery, and garlic and sauté until softened, about 5 minutes.

3. Stir in the xanthan gum and cook for 2 minutes.

4. Stir in the chicken broth and cook, stirring constantly, until the soup thickens, about 5 minutes.

5. Stir in the lobster meat, shrimp, cream, and thyme.

6. Cook, stirring occasionally, until the soup is heated through, about 10 minutes. Season with salt and pepper.

7. Divide among four bowls, top with the chives, and serve.

TIP: Xanthan gum is a keto-friendly thickening agent, similar in use to cornstarch. You can find it in the baking aisle of most grocery chains.

PER SERVING (¼ RECIPE): Calories: 417; Total Fat: 32g; Protein: 26g; Total Carbs: 6g; Fiber: 1g; Net Carbs: 5g
MACROS: Fat: 70% / Protein: 25% / Carbs: 5%

Beef Stroganoff

`ONE PAN` `GLUTEN-FREE`

You won't want to miss out on this creamy yet bold flavor combination, originally invented by a French chef in 1891.

SERVES 4
PREP TIME: 10 MINUTES
COOK TIME: 25 MINUTES

1 pound beef tenderloin or sirloin steak, cut into strips

Salt

Freshly ground black pepper

2 tablespoons butter, ghee, or butter-flavored coconut oil, divided

¼ cup sliced onions

1 cup sliced button mushrooms

1 garlic clove, minced

2 tablespoons almond flour

1½ cups Basic Broth, Beef Variation (page 180) or store-bought beef broth

2 tablespoons whole milk, plain Greek yogurt

1 teaspoon tamari

½ teaspoon Dijon mustard

½ teaspoon smoked paprika

⅛ teaspoon freshly squeezed lemon juice

⅛ teaspoon erythritol

Dash sugar-free hot sauce

1½ cups cooked shirataki noodles, well drained, or other cooked vegetable noodles

Chopped fresh parsley, for garnish (optional)

1. Season the beef with salt and pepper.

2. In a large, shallow skillet, melt 1 tablespoon of butter over medium-high heat. Add the beef and brown on both sides, 2 to 4 minutes total. Remove the beef from the pan and set aside.

3. In the same skillet, melt the remaining 1 tablespoon of butter, then add the onion, mushrooms, and garlic. Cook the vegetables for 4 minutes, then add the almond flour and stir to combine evenly.

4. Stir in the beef broth, reduce the heat to low, and continue stirring until thickened, 3 to 5 minutes.

5. Add the yogurt, tamari, mustard, paprika, lemon juice, erythritol, and hot sauce. Stir everything together again, then return the beef to the pan and let simmer for 5 to 8 minutes or until the beef is browned and juicy.

CONTINUED >>

6. Either add the shirataki noodles to the skillet and toss to combine with the sauce, or divide the noodles among 4 bowls and pour the sauce over them. Top with parsley (if using).

TIP: Don't be scared to mix it up and use another cut of meat if you're not feeling the beef. Chicken tenderloin is a great option, or you can even use whitefish such as halibut or swordfish.

PER SERVING (¼ RECIPE): Calories: 294; Total Fat: 20g; Protein: 25g; Total Carbs: 2g; Fiber: 1g; Net Carbs: 1g
MACROS: Fat: 61% / Protein: 36% / Carbs: 3%

Thai-Inspired Coconut Vegetable Soup

30-MINUTE | **ONE POT** | **GLUTEN-FREE** | **NUT-FREE** | **VEGAN**

If you've ever been to a Thai food restaurant, you'll probably recognize this take on tom yum soup. This recipe is the vegan keto version of the classic Thai dish. For a lighter version of this soup, omit the coconut cream. A good substitute is half an avocado to ensure you're getting plenty of healthy fat.

SERVES 4
PREP TIME: 10 MINUTES
COOK TIME: 20 MINUTES

8 cups Basic Broth (page 180) or store-bought vegetable broth

1 teaspoon ground ginger

2 garlic cloves, diced

1 lime, zested and cut into wedges

1 cup full-fat coconut cream

1 cup sliced mushrooms

1 tomato, coarsely chopped

½ medium yellow onion, coarsely chopped

1 cup coarsely chopped broccoli florets

1 cup coarsely chopped cauliflower florets

1 cup chopped fresh cilantro, for garnish (optional)

1. In a large stockpot, combine the broth, ginger, garlic, and lime zest. Bring to a simmer over medium heat.

2. Pour in the coconut cream, followed by the mushrooms, tomato, onion, broccoli, and cauliflower. Simmer until the vegetables are tender, about 15 minutes.

3. Remove the pot from the heat and serve the soup garnished with the cilantro (if using) and lime wedges.

PER SERVING (¼ RECIPE): Calories: 233; Total Fat: 21g; Protein: 5g; Total Carbs: 11g; Fiber: 3g; Net Carbs: 8g
MACROS: Fat: 76% / Protein: 6% / Carbs: 18%

Chicken Ramen Soup

DAIRY-FREE **GLUTEN-FREE** **NUT-FREE**

Traditional Japanese ramen includes broth, meat, vegetables, and non-keto-friendly noodles. This recipe packs the same savory punch as the classic soup but replaces the starchy noodles with shirataki noodles, which are made of vegetables. If you cannot find coconut aminos, use low-sodium soy sauce, but be aware that the recipe will no longer be gluten-free.

SERVES 4
PREP TIME: 25 MINUTES
COOK TIME: 30 MINUTES

2 (7-ounce) packages shirataki noodles

4 ounces shiitake mushrooms

1 teaspoon avocado oil

½ teaspoon sea salt

1 tablespoon olive oil

3½ tablespoons shredded carrots

2 garlic cloves, minced

¼ teaspoon ground ginger

4 cups Basic Broth, Chicken Variation (page 180) or store-bought chicken broth

2 cups shredded cooked chicken

2½ tablespoons coconut aminos

4 soft-boiled eggs, halved

1 scallion, white part only, diced (optional)

Hot sauce (optional)

1. Preheat the oven to 400°F. Line a baking sheet with paper towels. Line a second baking sheet with parchment paper.

2. Rinse and drain the noodles thoroughly. Place them on the paper towel–lined baking sheet and cover with more paper towels. Gently press to soak up the water. Discard the top layer of paper towels and let the noodles air-dry for 20 minutes.

3. Meanwhile, place the mushrooms (stems and caps) on the parchment paper–lined baking sheet and drizzle evenly with the avocado oil. Sprinkle with the salt. Bake for 20 minutes, until browned. Set aside.

4. While the mushrooms are baking, in a large saucepan, heat the olive oil over medium heat. Add the carrots, garlic, and ginger. Cook until fragrant, 1 to 2 minutes, stirring frequently so the garlic does not burn.

5. Add the noodles and stir-fry for another 2 to 3 minutes.

6. Add the chicken broth, chicken, and coconut aminos. Bring the mixture to a boil, then reduce the heat to low and simmer for 5 minutes, until the flavors have melded.

7. Divide the soup among four bowls. Top each bowl of ramen equally with a halved egg, mushrooms, and scallions (if using). Drizzle with hot sauce (if using).

TIP: Swap the chicken version of Basic Broth (page 180) for the beef variation and trade the chicken for 1 pound of cooked, sliced flank steak. Or go vegetarian by using the vegetable broth variation and 2 cups of bok choy instead of chicken.

PER SERVING (1 CUP): Calories: 235; Total Fat: 12g; Protein: 26g; Total Carbs: 4g; Fiber: 1g; Net Carbs: 3g
MACROS: Fat: 47% / Protein: 47% / Carbs: 6%

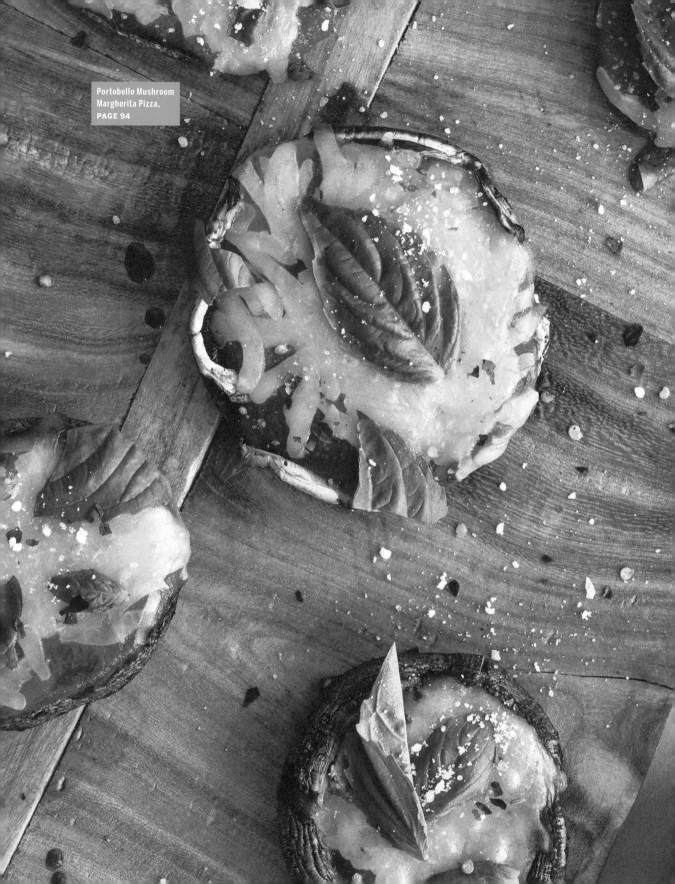

Portobello Mushroom
Margherita Pizza,
PAGE 94

Vegetable Mains and Sides

Roasted Veggies

5-INGREDIENT **30-MINUTE** **GLUTEN-FREE** **NUT-FREE** **VEGAN**

You can roast pretty much any vegetable. Cauliflower, broccoli, and Brussels sprouts are especially delicious when cooked this way, but feel free to experiment with your favorites. Just make sure you chop the vegetables into pieces that are about the same size so they roast evenly.

SERVES 4
PREP TIME: 5 MINUTES
COOK TIME: 25 MINUTES

1 cup cauliflower florets

1 cup broccoli florets

1 cup Brussels sprouts, trimmed and halved

2 tablespoons extra-virgin olive oil

Salt

Freshly ground black pepper

1. Preheat the oven to 425°F.

2. In a medium bowl, toss the cauliflower, broccoli, and Brussels sprouts with the olive oil, and season with salt and pepper.

3. On a baking sheet, spread the vegetables in a single layer. Be careful not to crowd them or the vegetables might steam rather than roast.

4. Cook the vegetables for 20 to 25 minutes, stirring once about halfway through, until browned and slightly crisp.

5. Sprinkle with a little more salt and pepper before serving.

TIP: Another great mix of vegetables is green beans, zucchini, asparagus, and bell peppers. This mix needs to roast for only about 15 minutes—otherwise, prepare it the same way.

PER SERVING (¼ SERVING): Calories: 83; Total Fat: 7g; Protein: 2g; Total Carbs: 5g; Fiber: 2g; Net Carbs: 3g
MACROS: Fat: 74% / Protein: 6% / Carbs: 20%

Cauliflower Mash

5-INGREDIENT | 30-MINUTE | GLUTEN-FREE | NUT-FREE | VEGETARIAN

If you haven't tried cauliflower mash yet, be prepared to have your mind blown. Master this basic recipe and then experiment by adding fresh herbs, dried spices, or heavy cream. An unexpected (yet delicious) addition is grated horseradish.

SERVES 2
PREP TIME: 5 MINUTES
COOK TIME: 10 MINUTES

1 head cauliflower, cut into small florets (about 1½ cups)

2 tablespoons extra-virgin olive oil

2 tablespoons butter or ghee

Salt

Freshly ground black pepper

1. Bring a large pot of water to a boil over high heat.

2. Add the cauliflower florets and cook until very tender, 8 to 10 minutes. Drain and let cool slightly.

3. Transfer the cauliflower to a blender or food processor.

4. Add the oil and butter, and blend until smooth and creamy, stopping a few times to scrape down the sides of the blender or food processor bowl.

5. Season to taste with salt and pepper. Serve immediately.

TIP: Top with a dollop of compound butter, such as one flavored with garlic and herbs.

PER SERVING (½ RECIPE): Calories: 274; Total Fat: 26g; Protein: 3g; Total Carbs: 7g; Fiber: 3g; Net Carbs: 4g
MACROS: Fat: 85% / Protein: 4% / Carbs: 11%

Pan-Roasted Green Beans

5-INGREDIENT | **30-MINUTE** | **ONE PAN** | **GLUTEN-FREE** | **VEGETARIAN**

It takes just a few ingredients to elevate green beans to star status; in this case, sliced almonds, Parmesan, garlic salt, and pepper do the trick. This dish is a family favorite and so easy to make, even with frozen green beans. Frozen beans are handy and can taste as good as fresh—just rinse them and pat them dry so they cook up crisp.

SERVES 4
PREP TIME: 5 MINUTES
COOK TIME: 15 MINUTES

3 tablespoons extra-virgin olive oil

1 (12-ounce) bag frozen green beans, rinsed and patted dry

1 teaspoon garlic salt

1 teaspoon freshly ground black pepper

¼ cup sliced almonds

¼ cup grated Parmesan cheese

1. In a skillet, heat the oil over medium heat until shimmering.

2. Add the green beans, garlic salt, and pepper and cook, stirring frequently and tossing to coat, for 10 to 12 minutes.

3. Increase the heat to high and keep moving the beans around until they begin to brown.

4. Sprinkle in the almonds and stir to combine.

5. Remove from the heat, sprinkle the Parmesan cheese on top, and serve.

TIP: Be sure to dry the beans well before putting them in the skillet so there's no additional moisture. To make this a full meal, add some chicken, sausage, or hamburger meat. Just be sure to add the additional carbs to your total.

PER SERVING (¼ RECIPE): Calories: 193; Total Fat: 16g; Protein: 6g; Total Carbs: 8g; Fiber: 3g; Net Carbs: 5g
MACROS: Fat: 72% / Protein: 12% / Carbs: 16%

Cauliflower Mac and "Cheese"

5-INGREDIENT · **30-MINUTE** · **GLUTEN-FREE** · **VEGAN**

Although a lot of people assume vegetables have more nutrition the deeper in color they are, cauliflower is jam-packed with essential vitamins and minerals. Vitamin K, which supports your bones, and vitamin C, which aids immune health and collagen production, are two shining stars in this vegetable. Paired with a silky butternut squash sauce, it's mac and cheese as you've never seen it before!

SERVES 2
PREP TIME: 5 MINUTES
COOK TIME: 15 MINUTES

1 small head cauliflower, coarsely chopped

1 batch Butternut Squash "Cheese" Sauce (page 185)

Salt

Freshly ground black pepper

Chopped fresh parsley, for serving (optional)

Sugar-free hot sauce, for serving (optional)

1. In a deep pot over medium heat, cover the cauliflower with about ¼ inch of water. Cover and steam for 5 to 7 minutes, until tender-crisp.

2. Turn off the heat and let the cauliflower continue to steam until easily pierced with a fork.

3. Meanwhile, in a saucepan, warm the "cheese" sauce over low heat for a few minutes.

4. Using a slotted spoon, remove the cauliflower from the pot and divide it between two bowls. Spoon or pour the cheese sauce evenly over the cauliflower and stir together.

5. Season with salt and pepper, sprinkle with parsley (if using), and top with hot sauce (if using).

PER SERVING (½ RECIPE): Calories: 343; Total Fat: 15g; Protein: 15g; Total Carbs: 37g; Fiber: 14g; Net Carbs: 23g
MACROS: Fat: 40% / Protein: 18% / Carbs: 42%

Sautéed Summer Squash

5-INGREDIENT **30-MINUTE** **ONE PAN** **GLUTEN-FREE** **VEGAN**

Summer squash is hugely versatile. You can eat it sliced, chopped, or spiralized. Plus, its flavor is mild enough that you can mix and match seasonings. Feel free to add different spices to this dish to make it your own.

SERVES 2
PREP TIME: 5 MINUTES
COOK TIME: 10 MINUTES

2 tablespoons avocado oil

1 zucchini, cut into half moons

1 yellow summer squash, cut into half moons

Salt

Freshly ground black pepper

2 teaspoons freshly grated Parmesan cheese (optional)

1. In a large skillet, heat the oil over medium heat until shimmering.

2. Add the zucchini and yellow squash in as even a layer as possible. It should sizzle as it hits the skillet. Sprinkle with salt and pepper.

3. Cook undisturbed for 2 minutes, until golden.

4. Give it a good stir, then cook for an additional 5 minutes, stirring occasionally, until the squash is tender.

5. Transfer to a bowl and sprinkle with the Parmesan cheese (if using).

PER SERVING (½ RECIPE): Calories: 162; Total Fat: 14g; Protein: 2g; Total Carbs: 7g; Fiber: 2g; Net Carbs: 5g
MACROS: Fat: 78% / Protein: 5% / Carbs: 17%

Wild Mushroom Tofu Ragù

ONE PAN **GLUTEN-FREE** **NUT-FREE** **VEGETARIAN**

Mushrooms have an earthy taste that complements the heavy cream, garlic, and thyme in this stew. You may think of herbs only in terms of flavor, but these little plants are also superfoods. Thyme, for instance, is high in volatile oils and flavonoids, as well as vitamin K and iron. Be generous with your thyme shaker, and your body will thank you.

SERVES 4
PREP TIME: 15 MINUTES
COOK TIME: 25 MINUTES

3 tablespoons extra-virgin olive oil

2 zucchini, diced

1 medium yellow onion, chopped

1 tablespoon minced garlic

1 pound assorted wild mushrooms, sliced

8 ounces extra-firm tofu, pressed

1 cup heavy (whipping) cream

½ cup Basic Broth (page 180) or store-bought vegetable broth

2 teaspoons chopped fresh thyme

Sea salt

Freshly ground black pepper

1. In a large skillet, heat the olive oil over medium-high heat.

2. Add the zucchini, onion, and garlic and sauté until tender, about 6 minutes.

3. Stir in the mushrooms and tofu and sauté until the liquid purges and the mushrooms caramelize, about 10 minutes.

4. Stir in the heavy cream, broth, and thyme and bring the ragù to a boil.

5. Reduce the heat to low and simmer until the sauce thickens, about 6 minutes.

6. Season with salt and pepper and serve.

TIP: For a vegan-friendly option, swap the heavy cream for the same amount of coconut milk and add a scoop of vegan protein powder. This will change the calories to 395 per serving and the macros to Fat: 71% / Protein: 20% / Carbs: 9%.

PER SERVING (¼ RECIPE): Calories: 416; Total Fat: 36g; Protein: 11g; Total Carbs: 17g; Fiber:5g; Net Carbs: 12g
MACROS: Fat: 76% / Protein: 9% / Carbs: 15%

Portobello Mushroom Margherita Pizza

5-INGREDIENT **30-MINUTE** **GLUTEN-FREE** **NUT-FREE** **VEGETARIAN**

Portobello mushrooms have a meaty texture that soaks up spices, herbs, and other flavorings like a sponge. It's no wonder they're a main course in many vegan and vegetarian restaurants. Mushrooms are a rare vegetable source of vitamin D and also contain high levels of potassium. The fats (cheese and olive oil) in this recipe help you absorb that all-important vitamin D.

SERVES 4
PREP TIME: 15 MINUTES
COOK TIME: 10 MINUTES

¾ cup extra-virgin olive oil

2 teaspoons minced garlic

6 large portobello
  mushrooms, stemmed

1½ cups canned tomato sauce

3 cups shredded
  mozzarella cheese

3 tablespoons chopped fresh
  basil, for garnish

TIP: If you're not vegetarian, pepperoni, Italian sausage, and prosciutto are delectable additions to these hearty pizzas. Meat will add protein and a few grams of fat to the dish.

1. Preheat the oven to broil. Line a baking sheet with aluminum foil and set aside.

2. In a medium bowl, stir together the olive oil and garlic, then add the mushrooms. Rub the oil all over the mushrooms and place them gill-side down on the prepared baking sheet.

3. Broil the mushrooms until they are tender, turning once, about 4 minutes total.

4. Remove the baking sheet from the oven and evenly divide the tomato sauce among the mushroom caps, spreading it on the gill side. Then top with the mozzarella cheese.

5. Return the sheet to the oven and broil the mushrooms until the cheese is melted and bubbly, 1 to 2 minutes.

6. Serve topped with the basil.

PER SERVING (1½ MUSHROOMS): Calories: 662; Total Fat: 60g; Protein: 22g; Total Carbs: 12g; Fiber: 3g; Net Carbs: 9g
MACROS: Fat: 80% / Protein: 14% / Carbs: 6%

Garlicky Broccoli Rabe with Artichokes

30-MINUTE GLUTEN-FREE NUT-FREE VEGAN

Broccoli rabe, or rapini, is packed with nutrients, including vitamins C and K, electrolytes, calcium, potassium, and dietary fiber, making it a great addition to your plate. You can use regular broccoli instead, but be sure to trim and finely slice the stalk and florets.

SERVES 4
PREP TIME: 5 MINUTES
COOK TIME: 15 MINUTES

2 pounds broccoli rabe

½ cup extra-virgin olive oil, divided

3 garlic cloves, finely minced

1 teaspoon salt

1 teaspoon red pepper flakes

1 (13.75-ounce) can artichoke hearts, drained and quartered

1 tablespoon water

2 tablespoons red wine vinegar

Freshly ground black pepper (optional)

1. Trim away any thick lower stems or yellow leaves from the broccoli rabe and discard. Cut into individual florets with a few inches of thin stem attached.

2. In a large skillet, heat ¼ cup of olive oil over medium-high heat. When it shimmers, add the trimmed broccoli, garlic, salt, and red pepper flakes and sauté for 5 minutes, until the broccoli begins to soften. Add the artichoke hearts and sauté for another 2 minutes until browned.

3. Add the water and reduce the heat to low. Cover and simmer until the broccoli stems are tender, 3 to 5 minutes.

4. In a small bowl, whisk together the remaining ¼ cup of olive oil and the vinegar. Drizzle over the broccoli and artichokes. Season with pepper (if using).

PER SERVING (¼ RECIPE): Calories: 385; Total Fat: 35g; Protein: 11g; Total Carbs: 18g; Fiber: 10g; Net Carbs: 8g
MACROS: Fat: 81% / Protein: 8% / Carbs: 11%

Green Vegetable Stir-Fry with Tofu

`ONE PAN` `GLUTEN-FREE` `NUT-FREE` `VEGAN`

If you have allergies, this stir-fry could be a wonderful substitute for seasonal allergy medication, because it's loaded with quercetin, a natural antihistamine.

SERVES 2
PREP TIME: 15 MINUTES
COOK TIME: 20 MINUTES

3 tablespoons avocado
   oil, divided

1 cup Brussels sprouts, trimmed
   and halved

½ medium white onion, diced

½ leek, white and light green
   parts diced

½ head green cabbage, diced

¼ cup water, plus more
   if needed

1 cup coarsely chopped spinach

½ cup coarsely chopped
   stemmed kale

8 ounces tofu, diced

2 teaspoons garlic powder

Salt

Freshly ground black pepper

½ avocado, pitted, peeled,
   and diced

MCT oil (optional)

1. In a large skillet or wok, heat 2 tablespoons of avocado oil over medium-high heat until shimmering. Add the Brussels sprouts, onion, leek, and cabbage and stir together.

2. Add the water and cover. Lower the heat to medium and cook for about 5 minutes.

3. Add the spinach and kale and cook for 3 minutes, stirring constantly, until the onion, leek, and cabbage are caramelized.

4. Add the tofu, then season with the garlic powder, salt, pepper, and the remaining 1 tablespoon of avocado oil.

5. Turn the heat back up to medium-high and cook for about 10 minutes, stirring constantly, until the tofu is caramelized on all sides. If you experience any burning, lower the heat and add 2 to 3 tablespoons of water.

6. Divide between two plates and sprinkle with the diced avocado. Feel free to drizzle MCT oil (if using) over the top for a little extra fat, if you wish.

TIP: Always make sure you purchase organic soy products, because soy is often genetically modified.

PER SERVING (½ RECIPE): Calories: 473; Total Fat: 33g; Protein: 17g; Total Carbs: 27g; Fiber: 12g; Net Carbs: 15g
MACROS: Fat: 63% / Protein: 15% / Carbs: 22%

Zucchini Noodles with Avocado-Kale Pesto

5-INGREDIENT | **30-MINUTE** | **ONE PAN** | **GLUTEN-FREE** | **VEGETARIAN**

Simple is best when you need a quick, satisfying meal. What's simpler than vegetable noodles tossed with flavor-packed pesto? You'll find spiralized zucchini in most grocery stores, and it keeps fresh for nearly a week in the refrigerator. Zucchini is rich in antioxidants such as beta-carotene and lutein, and it combines well with the avocado-rich pesto because the monounsaturated fats in avocado increase the absorption of fat-soluble beta-carotene.

SERVES 4
PREP TIME: 15 MINUTES
COOK TIME: 5 MINUTES

1 tablespoon extra-virgin olive oil

4 large zucchini, spiralized (or about 2 pounds if prepackaged)

¾ cup Avocado-Kale Pesto (page 188) or store-bought pesto

1 cup grated Parmesan cheese, for serving

1 tablespoon chopped fresh basil, for serving

1. In a large skillet, heat the olive oil over medium heat until shimmering.

2. Add the zucchini noodles and sauté until just heated through, about 4 minutes.

3. Add the pesto to the skillet and toss to coat.

4. Serve topped with the Parmesan cheese and basil.

TIP: If you wish, use basil pesto or sun-dried tomato pesto in place of the avocado-kale pesto. Most pesto is high in fat and moderately high in protein, so you should be fine on macros.

PER SERVING (¼ RECIPE): Calories: 297; Total Fat: 23g; Protein: 15g; Total Carbs: 9g; Fiber: 4g; Net Carbs: 5g
MACROS: Fat: 70% / Protein: 20% / Carbs: 10%

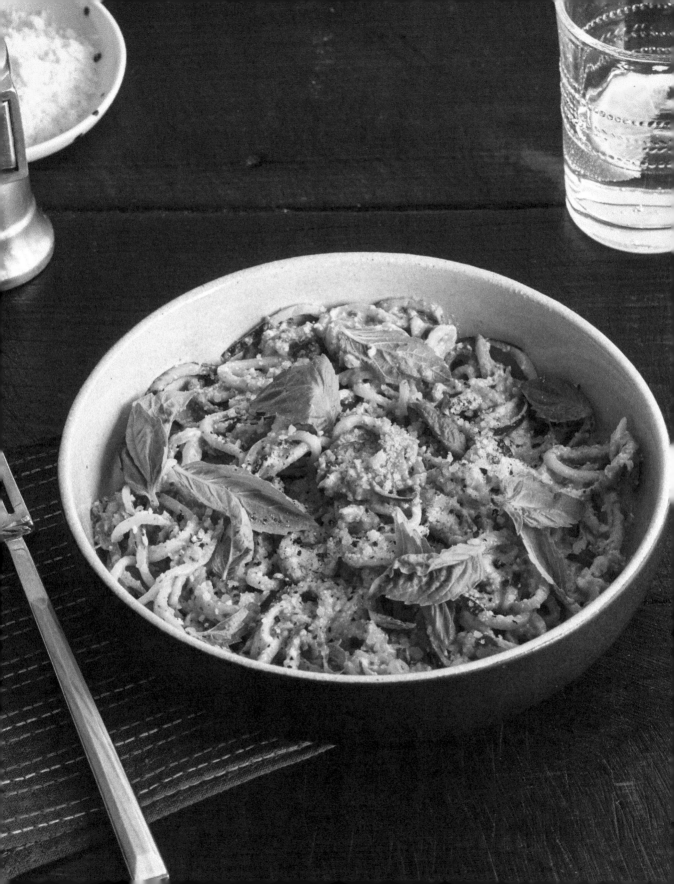

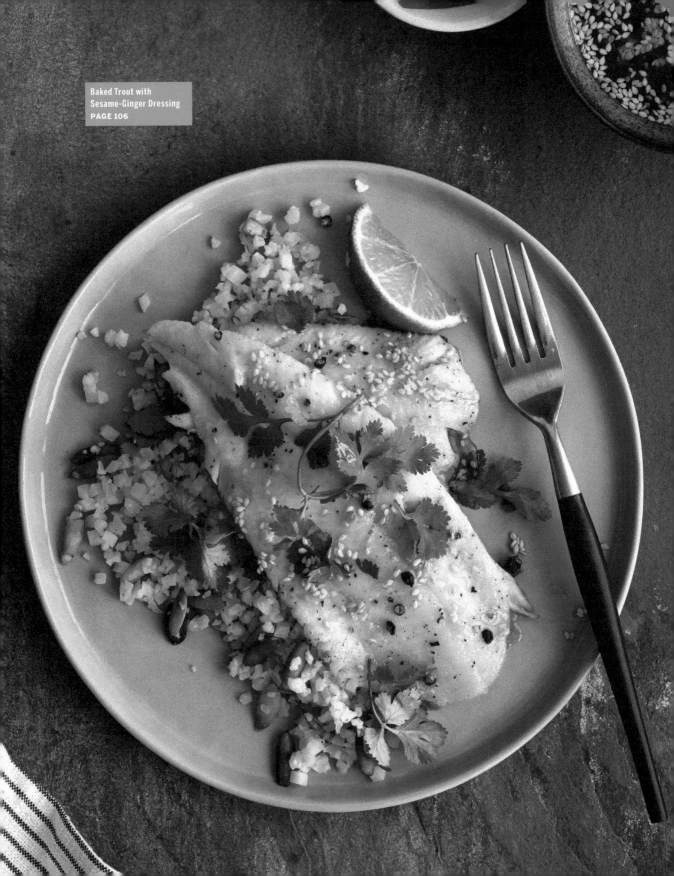

Baked Trout with
Sesame-Ginger Dressing
PAGE 106

Seafood

Tuna Melt

30-MINUTE | GLUTEN-FREE

A tuna melt is basically the marriage of tuna salad and a grilled cheese sandwich. Bread and celery provide a playful crunch to the soft sandwich interior. Easy to prep and easy to cook, this recipe is a great choice even on the busiest of days.

SERVES 2
PREP TIME: 10 MINUTES
COOK TIME: 5 MINUTES

2 (5-ounce) cans water-packed, solid white albacore tuna, drained

¼ cup plus 2 tablespoons Keto Mayonnaise (page 186) or store-bought mayonnaise

1 celery stalk, diced

1 tablespoon Dijon mustard

1 teaspoon freshly squeezed lemon juice

¼ teaspoon dried parsley

⅛ teaspoon freshly ground black pepper

2 batches 90-Second Bread (page 182)

4 slices cheddar cheese

1. Preheat the oven to broil. Line a baking sheet with parchment paper.

2. In a medium bowl, mix together the tuna, mayonnaise, celery, mustard, lemon juice, parsley, and pepper. Stir until thoroughly combined.

3. When the bread is cool enough to handle, slice each piece in half and toast.

4. Lay the 4 pieces of toast on the prepared baking sheet. Top each piece with an equal amount of tuna salad, followed by a slice of cheese.

5. Broil for 2 to 3 minutes or until the cheese has melted. Serve immediately. This dish does not store well, so halve the recipe if needed.

TIP: Adding veggies such as cooked spinach and a slice of tomato ups the flavor, texture, and nutrition of this tuna melt. Top the tuna salad with your vegetables of choice, then cover with the cheese before broiling.

PER SERVING (½ RECIPE): Calories: 956; Total Fat: 80g; Protein: 52g; Total Carbs: 7g; Fiber: 3g; Net Carbs: 4g
MACROS: Fat: 75% / Protein: 22% / Carbs: 3%

Fish Avocado Tacos

GLUTEN-FREE **NUT-FREE**

Cumin is the most prominent flavor in this recipe, and its peppery flavor pairs well with the salmon. It is high in iron and contains calcium, manganese, and magnesium—key minerals for supporting bone health.

SERVES 4
PREP TIME: 20 MINUTES
COOK TIME: 15 MINUTES

4 (4-ounce) salmon fillets

1 teaspoon ground cumin

⅛ teaspoon ground cayenne pepper

Sea salt

2 tablespoons extra-virgin olive oil

½ cup Keto Mayonnaise (page 186) or store-bought mayonnaise

¼ cup sour cream

Juice of 1 lime

1 teaspoon sriracha sauce

1 cup shredded cabbage

1 cup shredded celery root (celeriac)

1 carrot, shredded

4 large lettuce leaves

1 avocado, pitted, peeled, and diced

1 tablespoon finely chopped, fresh cilantro

1. Preheat the oven to 350°F.

2. Pat the salmon fillets dry with paper towels and place them in a single layer in a 9-by-9-inch baking dish.

3. Season the fish lightly with the cumin, cayenne, and salt.

4. Drizzle with the olive oil and bake for 12 to 15 minutes, until just cooked through.

5. While the fish is baking, in a medium bowl, stir the mayonnaise, sour cream, lime juice, and sriracha until well blended. Stir in the cabbage, celery root, and carrot until mixed.

6. When the fish is cooked, arrange the lettuce leaves on serving plates and place a fish fillet in the center of each.

7. Top with the slaw, avocado, and cilantro and serve.

TIP: Make the slaw topping up to 3 days ahead of time and store, sealed, in the refrigerator. Or use leftovers as a topping for pork, poultry, or other meals.

PER SERVING (¼ RECIPE): Calories: 660; Total Fat: 46g; Protein: 32g; Total Carbs: 36g; Fiber: 15g; Net Carbs: 21g
MACROS: Fat: 62% / Protein: 18% / Carbs: 20%

Salmon Cakes with Avocado

DAIRY-FREE GLUTEN-FREE

Make sure to look for wild-caught red salmon for these cakes, preferably sockeye. Unlike many seafood dishes, these cakes freeze well, making cooking a big batch for use in later meals a huge plus.

SERVES 4
PREP TIME: 15 MINUTES, PLUS 15 MINUTES TO REST
COOK TIME: 15 MINUTES

1 (14.5-ounce) can red salmon or 1 pound cooked skinless wild-caught salmon fillet

½ cup minced red onion

1 very ripe avocado, pitted, peeled, and mashed

1 large egg

2 tablespoons Keto Mayonnaise (page 186) or store-bought mayonnaise, plus more for serving

½ cup almond flour

1 to 2 teaspoons dried dill

1 teaspoon garlic powder

1 teaspoon salt

½ teaspoon smoked paprika

½ teaspoon freshly ground black pepper

Zest and juice of 1 lemon

¼ cup extra-virgin olive oil

1. Remove the spine, large bones, and pieces of skin from the salmon (don't worry about the small bones if using canned). Combine the salmon and red onion in a large bowl and, using a fork, break up any lumps.

2. Add the avocado, egg, and mayonnaise and combine well.

3. In a small bowl, whisk the almond flour, dill, garlic powder, salt, paprika, and pepper.

4. To the salmon, add the dry ingredient mixture plus the lemon zest and juice. Combine well.

5. Form into 8 small patties, about 2 inches in diameter, and place on a plate. Let rest for 15 minutes.

6. In a large, cast-iron skillet, heat the olive oil over medium heat until shimmering. Fry the patties until browned, 2 to 3 minutes per side.

7. Cover the skillet, reduce the heat to low, and cook another 6 to 8 minutes, or until the cakes are set in the center. Remove from the skillet and serve warm with additional mayonnaise.

TIP: These salmon cakes can be stored in the refrigerator or freezer for using on salads, crumbled in scrambled eggs, or for a quick high-protein snack.

PER SERVING (¼ RECIPE): Calories: 513; Total Fat: 40g; Protein: 30g; Total Carbs: 10g; Fiber: 5g; Net Carbs: 5g
MACROS: Fat: 68% / Protein: 24% / Carbs: 8%

Baked Trout with Sesame-Ginger Dressing

30-MINUTE **DAIRY-FREE** **GLUTEN-FREE** **NUT-FREE**

Trout is high in protein, omega-3 fatty acids, potassium, and B vitamins, which makes it a great choice for a healthy diet. Rainbow trout, you'll be glad to know, is one of the least contaminated farmed fish.

SERVES 4
PREP TIME: 10 MINUTES
COOK TIME: 15 MINUTES

4 (3-ounce) trout fillets

Sea salt

Freshly ground black pepper

¼ cup extra-virgin olive oil

2 tablespoons apple cider vinegar

1 tablespoon toasted sesame oil

1 tablespoon coconut aminos

1½ teaspoons peeled, grated, fresh ginger

½ teaspoon garlic powder

½ teaspoon toasted sesame seeds

1 tablespoon chopped fresh cilantro, for garnish

1 lime, quartered, for garnish

1. Preheat the oven to 400°F.

2. Pat the trout fillets dry with paper towels. Lightly season with salt and pepper and arrange in a single layer in a 9-by-9-inch baking dish.

3. In a medium bowl, whisk the olive oil, apple cider vinegar, sesame oil, coconut aminos, ginger, garlic powder, and sesame seeds until well emulsified.

4. Spoon 1 tablespoon of dressing onto each piece of fish.

5. Bake for 12 to 14 minutes, until the fish is just cooked through.

6. Spoon the remaining dressing over the fish and serve topped with the cilantro and lime wedges.

PER SERVING (¼ TROUT RECIPE): Calories: 129; Total Fat: 6g; Protein: 18g; Total Carbs: 1g; Fiber: 0g; Net Carbs: 1g
MACROS: Fat: 59% / Protein: 39% / Carbs: 2%

PER SERVING (1 TABLESPOON DRESSING): Calories: 153; Total Fat: 16g; Protein: 1g; Total Carbs: 1g; Fiber: 0g; Net Carbs: 1g
MACROS: Fat: 97% / Protein: 2% / Carbs: 1%

Shrimp in Creamy Pesto over Zoodles

30-MINUTE **GLUTEN-FREE**

This easy weeknight recipe is both indulgent and fresh. You can make this with chicken thighs as well, browning the thighs with the onions. Remove them before bringing the pesto and cheese to a simmer, then return them to the sauce until cooked through, about 20 minutes.

SERVES 4
PREP TIME: 10 MINUTES
COOK TIME: 10 MINUTES

1 pound shrimp, peeled and deveined

Salt

Freshly ground black pepper

2 tablespoons extra-virgin olive oil

½ small yellow onion, slivered

1 cup Avocado-Kale Pesto (page 188) or store-bought pesto

¾ cup crumbled goat or feta cheese, plus more for serving

6 cups zucchini noodles, from about 2 large zucchini, for serving

¼ cup chopped fresh flat-leaf Italian parsley, for garnish

1. In a bowl, season the shrimp with salt and pepper and set aside.

2. In a large skillet, heat the olive oil over medium-high heat. Add the onion and sauté until just golden, 5 to 6 minutes.

3. Reduce the heat to low and add the pesto and cheese, whisking to combine and melt the cheese. Bring to a low simmer and add the shrimp.

4. Cover and cook until the shrimp is cooked through and pink, another 3 to 4 minutes.

5. Serve warm over zucchini noodles, garnishing with chopped parsley and additional crumbled cheese.

PER SERVING (¼ RECIPE): Calories: 576; Total Fat: 46g; Protein: 35g; Total Carbs: 9g; Fiber: 3g; Net Carbs: 6g
MACROS: Fat: 71% / Protein: 23% / Carbs: 6%

Lobster "Mac" and Cheese

30-MINUTE | **ONE PAN** | **GLUTEN-FREE** | **NUT-FREE**

Creamy Brie cheese with lobster tail sautéed in butter may sound like something you would get at a fancy restaurant, but this dish is easy to prepare at home. It's definitely a splurge, though, so save it for a special occasion.

SERVES 1
PREP TIME: 10 MINUTES
COOK TIME: 20 MINUTES

1 (4-ounce) lobster tail

1 tablespoon salted butter

1 (8-ounce) bag frozen cauliflower florets, thawed and patted dry

Salt

Freshly ground black pepper

½ cup heavy cream

3 ounces Brie cheese, cubed

1 tablespoon chopped fresh chives, for garnish

1. Using kitchen shears or a sharp knife, carefully split the lobster tail in half lengthwise. Remove the tail meat and cut it into bite-size pieces.

2. In a medium pan, melt the butter over medium heat. Add the lobster and cook for about 3 minutes until the meat turns white and is almost fully cooked.

3. Add the cauliflower florets and season with salt and pepper. Cook for about 2 minutes, until warmed.

4. Add the heavy cream and cook for 2 minutes, stirring occasionally, until it has reduced by about half.

5. Reduce the heat to low and stir in the Brie a few cubes at a time until the sauce is smooth. Make sure the lobster and cauliflower are fully coated.

6. Garnish with the chives and serve.

TIP: Shrimp also works great in this dish. Look for raw peeled shrimp and cook them following the same instructions as the lobster. You can also substitute any cheese you like for the Brie. Try cheddar, provolone, or pepper Jack.

PER SERVING (ENTIRE RECIPE): Calories: 955; Total Fat: 81g; Protein: 46g; Total Carbs: 15g; Fiber: 10g; Net Carbs: 5g
MACROS: Fat: 74% / Protein: 20% / Carbs: 6%

Spicy Brown-Butter Shrimp

30-MINUTE **ONE POT** **GLUTEN-FREE** **NUT-FREE**

This dish takes only 20 minutes to prepare from start to finish. Serve it as an appetizer or alongside sautéed veggies or riced cauliflower as an entrée. Larger shrimp work best for this recipe—I recommend looking for a shrimp count of 21/25 per pound (see tip). Whatever size you're using, shrimp cooks very quickly, so make sure you have all your ingredients ready before you get cooking.

SERVES 2
PREP TIME: 10 MINUTES
COOK TIME: 10 MINUTES

2 tablespoons salted butter

1 pound shrimp, peeled and deveined, tails off

1 tablespoon minced garlic

4 tablespoons bourbon, rum, tequila, white wine, or chicken stock

1 jalapeño pepper, sliced

1 tablespoon chopped fresh parsley

1. In a medium pan, melt the butter over medium heat and let it foam. Once the butter begins to brown, add the shrimp and garlic.

2. Cook the shrimp for about 3 minutes per side, until pink and opaque.

3. Turn off the heat and carefully pour in the bourbon. It may flame up for a few seconds.

4. Once the flame dissipates, turn the heat back to medium and add the jalapeño and parsley. Serve immediately.

TIP: Shrimp are sold by the number of shrimp it takes to weigh 1 pound. A count of 21/25 means you'll get somewhere between 21 and 25 shrimp in a pound. Larger shrimp will be labeled 16/20 and smaller shrimp will be labelled 31/40. Words like jumbo, medium, and extra-large don't have any real regulation and will vary in meaning from brand to brand.

PER SERVING (½ RECIPE): Calories: 304; Total Fat: 13g; Protein: 46g; Total Carbs: 2g; Fiber: 0g; Net Carbs: 2g
MACROS: Fat: 37% / Protein: 61% / Carbs: 2%

Shrimp à la Vodka Pasta

30-MINUTE | **ONE POT** | **GLUTEN-FREE** | **NUT-FREE**

When buying marinara, be sure to check the labels for added sugar. Look for types that only have tomatoes, onions, garlic, olive oil, salt, pepper, and oregano. Make sure to rinse the hearts of palm noodles under cold water for 30 seconds to 1 minute and drain well afterward. This will remove any acidic flavor from the canning process.

SERVES 2
PREP TIME: 10 MINUTES
COOK TIME: 20 MINUTES

1 tablespoon olive oil

1 pound shrimp, peeled and deveined, tails off

1 tablespoon minced garlic

Salt

Freshly ground black pepper

4 tablespoons vodka

1 (14-ounce) package hearts of palm noodles, rinsed and drained (see tip)

¼ cup heavy (whipping) cream

¼ cup no-sugar-added marinara sauce

2 tablespoons chopped fresh basil, for garnish

Grated Parmesan cheese, for garnish

TIP: Hearts of palm noodles are pretty new in the keto world, but you can find them at many national grocery chains. If you can't find them, substitute zoodles or shirataki noodles.

1. In a medium pan, heat the oil over medium heat until shimmering. Add the shrimp and cook for 3 minutes per side, until pink and nearly opaque. Add the garlic, and salt and pepper to taste.

2. Pour in the vodka and cook for 1 minute, until the alcohol has burned off. Once the shrimp are fully cooked, remove them from the pan and set aside.

3. Add the hearts of palm noodles to the pan and cook for 3 to 4 minutes, until any excess water has cooked off.

4. Pour in the heavy cream and simmer for 2 minutes, stirring occasionally, until the cream begins to thicken. Add the marinara sauce and stir to incorporate. Toss the noodles in the sauce until they are fully coated.

5. Return the shrimp to the pan and cook just long enough to warm it through. Garnish with the basil and Parmesan cheese.

PER SERVING (½ RECIPE): Calories: 488; Total Fat: 19g; Protein: 53g; Total Carbs: 15g; Fiber: 6g; Net Carbs: 9g
MACROS: Fat: 39% / Protein: 47% / Carbs: 14%

Crispy-Skin Salmon

5-INGREDIENT · **30-MINUTE** · **DAIRY-FREE** · **GLUTEN-FREE** · **NUT-FREE**

Salmon skin contains the highest amounts of omega-3 fatty acids on the fish. Omega-3s are beneficial for every aspect of heart health and are essential for brain function and cell growth. Be sure to buy wild-caught salmon to reduce the risk of the fish being contaminated by pollutants.

SERVES 2
PREP TIME: 5 MINUTES
COOK TIME: 10 MINUTES

2 (6-ounce) skin-on salmon fillets

½ teaspoon salt

4 teaspoons coconut aminos

1. Pat the salmon dry, then sprinkle the skin side with salt (this will help absorb excess moisture from the skin).

2. Heat a large skillet over medium heat.

3. Place the salmon skin-side down in the skillet. Cook for about 6 minutes.

4. Reduce the heat and pour the coconut aminos over the top of the salmon.

5. Flip the salmon carefully and cook for 1 to 2 more minutes, until the internal temperature reaches 130°F for medium or 145°F for well done.

TIP: For more flavor, mix in 2 teaspoons of grated fresh ginger to the coconut aminos.

PER SERVING (½ RECIPE): Calories: 239; Total Fat: 11g; Protein: 33g; Total Carbs: 2g; Fiber: 0g; Net Carbs: 2g
MACROS: Fat: 40%; Protein: 59%; Carbs: 1%

Bacon-Wrapped Scallops with Sweet Balsamic Sauce

5-INGREDIENT | DAIRY-FREE | GLUTEN-FREE | NUT-FREE

Scallops are rich in omega-3 fatty acids, vitamin B_{12}, and antioxidants, which help improve cardiovascular function and lower cholesterol levels. They also contain minerals such as potassium and magnesium. But you'll love this easy dish because it tastes so decadent.

SERVES 2
PREP TIME: 5 MINUTES
COOK TIME: 30 MINUTES

8 slices bacon

4 teaspoons balsamic vinegar

4 teaspoons coconut aminos

8 medium sea scallops (about 6 ounces)

2 tablespoons coconut oil

1. Preheat the oven to 360°F. Line a baking sheet with parchment paper.

2. Place the bacon on the baking sheet, cook for 10 minutes, then flip and cook for an additional 6 minutes. Transfer the bacon slices to a paper towel–lined plate. (You want the bacon to still be flexible enough to wrap around the scallops.)

3. In a small saucepan, heat the balsamic vinegar and coconut aminos over medium heat until bubbling. Reduce the heat and let simmer for 5 minutes, until reduced.

4. Pat the scallops dry and wrap one slice of bacon around the circular edge of each scallop, folding the bacon down so that the scallop surface will touch the skillet. Spear each scallop with a toothpick to secure the bacon around it.

5. In a large skillet, heat the coconut oil over high heat until shimmering.

6. Gently add the scallops, flat-side down, to the skillet, making sure you don't overcrowd the pan. Cook for 2 to 3 minutes on each side, until golden.

7. Transfer the scallops to a plate and drizzle with the balsamic sauce. Serve.

TIP: Try to use thinly sliced bacon with a thin width for best results. Also, don't overcook the scallops or they will get tough and chewy.

PER SERVING (½ RECIPE): Calories: 447; Total Fat: 28g; Protein: 40g; Total Carbs: 6g; Fiber: 0g; Net Carbs: 6g
MACROS: Fat: 57% / Protein: 37% / Carbs: 6%

Fish Coconut Curry

ONE PAN **GLUTEN-FREE** **NUT-FREE**

The quality of a fish stew depends, in large part, on the type of fish used. The calorie, fat, and protein levels will vary in this recipe as you vary your fish choices. Salmon was used in the calculations here.

SERVES 4
PREP TIME: 15 MINUTES
COOK TIME: 30 MINUTES

¼ cup coconut oil

1 medium yellow onion, chopped

1 tablespoon minced garlic

1 tablespoon minced jalapeño pepper

1 tablespoon peeled, grated fresh ginger

1 cup diced eggplant

2 zucchini, diced

1½ tablespoons curry powder

½ teaspoon ground cumin

1 cup heavy (whipping) cream

1 cup Basic Broth, Chicken Variation (page 180) or store-bought chicken broth

2 cups green beans, cut into 1-inch pieces

1 pound firm fish, cut into 1-inch chunks

1 cup baby spinach

1. In a large saucepan, heat the coconut oil over medium-high heat until shimmering. Add the onion, garlic, jalapeño, and ginger and sauté for about 5 minutes, until softened. Add the eggplant and zucchini and sauté for 5 minutes until they're beginning to soften.

2. Stir in the curry powder and cumin and sauté for about 2 minutes until very fragrant. Stir in the heavy cream and chicken broth and bring the liquid to a boil.

3. Reduce the heat to low and simmer for about 5 minutes until the vegetables are tender.

4. Stir in the green beans and fish and simmer for 8 to 10 minutes, until the fish is cooked through.

5. Remove from the heat, stir in the spinach, and let the curry stand for 5 minutes to wilt the spinach. Serve.

TIP: Swap an equal amount of pressed, diced tofu for the fish. Sauté the tofu in coconut oil until crispy (in step 1) and transfer it to a plate. Return the tofu to the pan in step 4 and follow the directions as written.

PER SERVING (¼ RECIPE): Calories: 465; Total Fat: 37g; Protein: 22g; Total Carbs: 15g; Fiber: 6g; Net Carbs: 9g
MACROS: Fat: 70% / Protein: 19% / Carbs: 11%

Ahi Tuna Poke

30-MINUTE | ONE BOWL | DAIRY-FREE | NUT-FREE

If you enjoy sushi and sashimi, make your own at home in a flash. This dish is perfect as an appetizer, light meal, or party tray. If you want to kick it up a notch, add some red pepper flakes or chili sauce. It's also delicious with chunks of avocado mixed in. Just be sure to add the additional carbs to your total carb count.

SERVES 4
PREP TIME: 10 MINUTES

3 scallions, white and green parts, diced

½ cup soy sauce or tamari

2 teaspoons toasted sesame oil

1 tablespoon sesame seeds

1 teaspoon garlic powder

1 teaspoon salt

¼ teaspoon ground ginger

2 pounds fresh ahi tuna, cut into ½-inch cubes

1. In a medium bowl, mix the scallions, soy sauce, sesame oil, sesame seeds, garlic powder, salt, and ginger.

2. Combine the soy sauce mixture with the tuna and toss well. Serve immediately.

TIP: If not serving immediately, store the tuna and the soy sauce mixture separately in the refrigerator until ready to serve.

PER SERVING (¼ RECIPE): Calories: 241; Total Fat: 9g; Protein: 38g; Carbs: 2g; Fiber: 1g; Net Carbs: 1g
MACROS: Fat: 34% / Protein: 63 % / Carbs: 3%

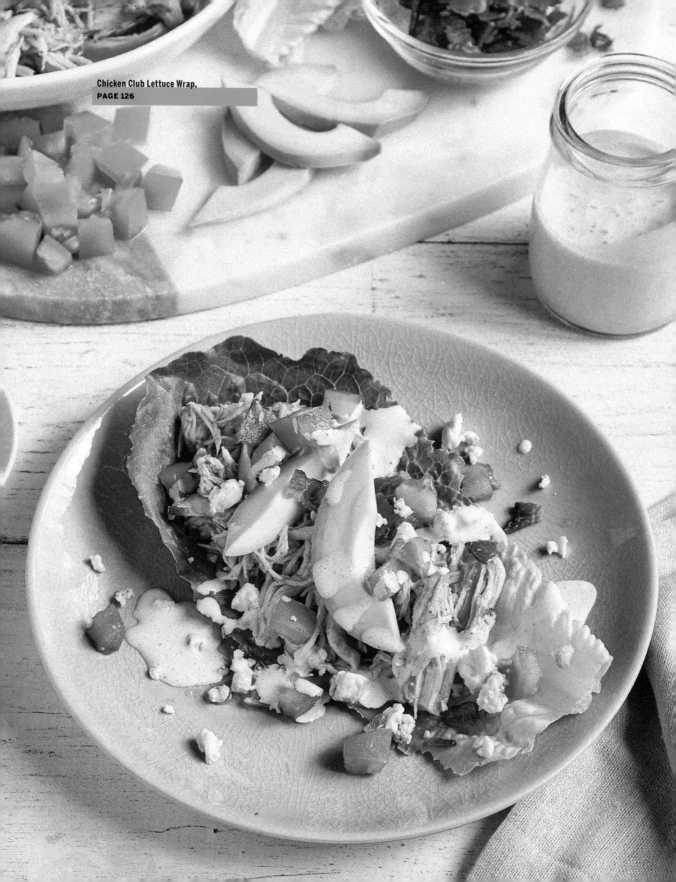

Chicken Club Lettuce Wrap,
PAGE 126

Poultry

Crispy Fried Chicken Bites

DAIRY-FREE **GLUTEN-FREE** **NUT-FREE**

Dip these chicken bites in your favorite keto-friendly sauce, such as Ranch Dressing (page 187) or sugar-free barbecue sauce. Marinating the chicken ahead of time adds extra flavor and helps the crushed pork rinds adhere to the chicken. Blitz the rinds in the food processor or put in a plastic bag and smash with a can.

SERVES 2
PREP TIME: 15 MINUTES, PLUS 30 MINUTES TO MARINATE
COOK TIME: 35 MINUTES

1 large egg

1 tablespoon Keto Mayonnaise (page 186) or store-bought mayonnaise

1 tablespoon Dijon mustard

½ teaspoon smoked paprika

½ teaspoon onion powder

½ teaspoon garlic powder

½ teaspoon freshly ground black pepper

¼ teaspoon salt

1 pound boneless, skinless chicken breast, cut into 2-inch pieces

1 cup crushed pork rinds

Avocado oil, for greasing

1. Preheat the oven to 450°F.

2. In a large mixing bowl, combine the egg, mayonnaise, mustard, smoked paprika, onion powder, garlic powder, pepper, and salt. Whisk until smooth.

3. Add the chicken and mix to completely coat. Cover and marinate in the refrigerator for 30 minutes.

4. Pour the crushed rinds into a bowl. Grease a baking sheet lightly with avocado oil.

5. One at a time, drop the chicken pieces into the pork rinds and toss to coat, pressing the crumbs gently into the chicken to adhere. Place each chicken bite on the prepared baking sheet.

6. Bake for 30 to 35 minutes, flipping the bites once after 15 minutes, until crispy and golden brown.

TIP: Make these in an air fryer. Put the chicken bites in the basket or tray, making sure not to crowd them too closely together, and cook at 400°F for about 30 minutes, flipping halfway through cooking.

PER SERVING (½ RECIPE): Calories: 466; Total Fat: 23g; Protein: 59g; Total Carbs: 2g; Fiber: 0g; Net Carbs: 2g
MACROS: Fat: 44% / Protein: 54% / Carbs: 2%

Caribbean Jerk Chicken Tenders with Creamy Mustard Sauce

DAIRY-FREE **GLUTEN-FREE** **NUT-FREE**

You don't always need to bread chicken tenders and fry them in oil to make them taste good. These Caribbean jerk tenders are baked in the oven, making them a fantastic low-carb, low-calorie option that's loaded with flavor. You can marinate the chicken overnight for a quick next-day meal, or cook the tenders in advance and use them as a salad topper drizzled with the mustard sauce for dressing.

SERVES 2
PREP TIME: 10 MINUTES, PLUS 30 MINUTES TO MARINATE
COOK TIME: 25 MINUTES

- 1 pound boneless skinless chicken breasts, cut into 1-inch-thick strips
- 1 tablespoon avocado oil
- 1 tablespoon Caribbean jerk seasoning, plus 1 teaspoon
- ¼ cup Keto Mayonnaise (page 186) or store-bought mayonnaise
- ¼ cup Dijon mustard
- 2 tablespoons powdered allulose (see tip)
- ¼ cup thinly sliced scallions, white and green parts, for serving

1. In a medium bowl, toss the chicken strips with the avocado oil and 1 tablespoon of jerk seasoning. Cover and marinate in the refrigerator for 30 minutes.

2. Preheat the oven to 425°F.

3. Lay the chicken strips on a baking sheet and bake for 20 minutes, until they reach an internal temperature of 165°F.

4. While the chicken is baking, prepare the dipping sauce. In a small bowl, combine the mayonnaise, mustard, allulose, and remaining 1 teaspoon of jerk seasoning.

5. Garnish the chicken tenders with the scallions and serve with the creamy mustard sauce.

TIP: These chicken tenders are even better when cooked on the grill (or grill pan). The charred flavor really elevates the Caribbean jerk flavor. Grill the strips for about 5 minutes per side until they reach an internal temperature of 165°F.

TIP: Allulose is a type of sugar found in jackfruit, figs, and raisins that the body does not metabolize into glucose. This means it doesn't get absorbed into the blood and cause a sugar spike the way granulated sugar does. Allulose is keto-friendly and it's available online and at national retailers such as Walmart and Target.

PER SERVING (½ RECIPE): Calories: 544; Total Fat: 35g; Protein: 53g; Total Carbs: 3g; Fiber: 2g; Net Carbs: 1g
MACROS: Fat: 57% / Protein: 41% / Carbs: 2%

Sesame Chicken Lettuce Cups

DAIRY-FREE **NUT-FREE**

These lettuce cups are fun to make and a great recipe for your regular rotation. Marinate the chicken up to 24 hours ahead, then simply sauté and serve with crispy napa cabbage leaves.

SERVES 2
PREP TIME: 10 MINUTES, PLUS 30 MINUTES TO MARINATE
COOK TIME: 10 MINUTES

1 pound boneless skinless chicken thighs, quartered

2 tablespoons soy sauce or coconut aminos

Zest and juice of 1 lime

1 tablespoon toasted sesame oil

2 teaspoons sriracha

1 teaspoon peeled, minced fresh ginger

1 teaspoon minced garlic

½ teaspoon five-spice seasoning

½ cup thinly sliced scallions, white and green parts separated

2 teaspoons sesame seeds

½ head napa cabbage

TIP: If you can't find napa cabbage, substitute red cabbage, romaine, Bibb, or iceberg lettuce.

1. Put the chicken in a food processor. Pulse for about 15 seconds, until the chicken is minced into very small chunks (slightly larger than ground chicken).

2. Transfer the chicken to a large bowl and add the soy sauce, lime zest and juice, sesame oil, sriracha, ginger, garlic, and five-spice seasoning. Mix well. Cover and marinate in the refrigerator for 30 minutes or up to 24 hours.

3. Set a medium skillet over high heat. Once hot, transfer the marinated chicken into the skillet. Using a wooden spoon or spatula, spread the chicken in an even layer, then cook undisturbed for 2 minutes, until golden. Stir.

4. Add the scallion white parts and continue to sauté for 2 to 3 minutes, until cooked through. Remove from the heat.

5. Garnish with the scallion greens and sesame seeds. Serve in cabbage leaves.

PER SERVING (½ RECIPE): Calories: 420; Total Fat: 15g; Protein: 56g; Total Carbs: 16g; Fiber: 6g; Net Carbs: 10g
MACROS: Fat: 31% / Protein: 55% / Carbs: 14%

Black and Blue Chicken Thighs

ONE PAN **GLUTEN-FREE** **NUT-FREE**

This simple recipe hits every part of your taste buds—spicy Cajun seasoning on smoky blackened chicken thighs, contrasted with creamy, melted blue cheese, salty bacon, and fresh tomatoes. Plus, you can make it all in one pan. If you don't like blue cheese, you can substitute Monterey Jack, Swiss, mozzarella, or Brie cheese.

SERVES 2
PREP TIME: 10 MINUTES, PLUS 30 MINUTES TO MARINATE
COOK TIME: 15 MINUTES

1 pound boneless, skinless chicken thighs

1 tablespoon Cajun seasoning

1 tablespoon avocado oil

½ cup crumbled blue cheese

¼ cup chopped cooked bacon

¼ cup diced tomatoes

¼ cup thinly sliced scallions, white and green parts

1. Trim any excess fat from the chicken thighs and sprinkle both sides with the Cajun seasoning. Cover and marinate in the refrigerator for 30 minutes.

2. Preheat the oven to broil.

3. In a medium, oven-safe skillet, heat the oil over high heat until shimmering. Add the chicken and sear for about 3 minutes per side, until blackened.

4. Sprinkle the chicken with the cheese, bacon, and tomatoes. Transfer the skillet to the oven and broil for 3 to 5 minutes until the cheese has melted.

5. Garnish with the scallions and serve alongside your favorite vegetables.

TIP: If you want to lower the calorie count of this recipe, use chicken breasts instead of thighs. Use a rolling pin or meat mallet to even out the thickness of the chicken breasts so they cook evenly. You can also slice the chicken breast into chicken tenders.

PER SERVING (½ RECIPE): Calories: 530; Total Fat: 31g; Protein: 57g; Total Carbs: 3g; Fiber: 1g; Net Carbs: 2g
MACROS: Fat: 53% / Protein: 45 % / Carbs: 2%

Bacon-Wrapped Barbecue Turkey Meatballs

GLUTEN-FREE   NUT-FREE

Bacon-wrapped turkey meatballs are low in carbs but packed with protein, making them a great keto option for an appetizer or full meal. This recipe also works with ground chicken if you prefer. Make sure to use lean ground turkey.

MAKES 20 MEATBALLS
PREP TIME: 15 MINUTES
COOK TIME: 30 MINUTES

1 pound 93% lean ground turkey

½ cup shredded cheddar cheese

¼ cup coconut flour

1 tablespoon barbecue spice rub

1 large egg

2 tablespoons dried, minced onion

10 slices bacon, halved crosswise

½ cup sugar-free barbecue sauce

¼ cup thinly sliced scallions, green part only

¼ cup Ranch Dressing (page 187) or store-bought ranch dressing

1. Preheat the oven to 425°F.

2. In a large bowl, combine the turkey, cheese, coconut flour, barbecue rub, egg, and dried onion. Mix just until combined (don't overmix or you'll have tough meatballs).

3. Form the mixture into 2-ounce meatballs (about the size of a golf ball). Wrap each meatball with a half slice of bacon and secure with a toothpick. Transfer to a large baking dish.

4. Bake for 25 minutes, until the turkey is cooked through and the bacon has browned. Remove from the oven.

5. Increase the oven to broil. Brush the meatballs liberally with the barbecue sauce.

6. Return to the oven and broil for 2 minutes, or until caramelized.

7. Top with the scallions and serve with ranch dressing for dipping.

TIP: For sauces, try Sweet Baby Ray's, Kinder's, or AlternaSweets. For dry rubs, check out Dan-O's or Spiceology's Salt Pepper Garlic blend. Always review the labels to check the sugar content.

PER SERVING (5 MEATBALLS): Calories: 525; Total Fat: 34g; Protein: 37g; Total Carbs: 13g; Fiber: 1g; Net Carbs: 12g
MACROS: Fat: 59% / Protein: 30% / Carbs: 11%

Chicken Club Lettuce Wrap

30-MINUTE | **ONE BOWL** | **GLUTEN-FREE** | **NUT-FREE**

This lettuce wrap is a great alternative to what you can get at the fast-food drive-through, and so easy to put together. Feel free to use any leftover chicken you have. This recipe is another great example of why you should keep a supply of Ranch Dressing (page 187) in your refrigerator.

SERVES 4
PREP TIME: 5 MINUTES

2 cups shredded cooked chicken (from 1 store-bought rotisserie chicken)

1 tomato, diced

1 avocado, pitted, peeled, and sliced

6 slices cooked bacon, crumbled

4 tablespoons crumbled blue cheese

8 romaine lettuce leaves

Salt

Freshly ground black pepper

½ cup Ranch Dressing (page 187) or store-bought ranch dressing

1. Divide the chicken, tomato, avocado, bacon, and cheese evenly among the lettuce leaves. Season with salt and pepper.

2. Drizzle the ranch dressing over each lettuce wrap; serve cold.

PER SERVING (¼ RECIPE): Calories: 405; Total Fat: 29g; Protein: 26g; Total Carbs: 9g; Fiber: 4g; Net Carbs: 5g
MACROS: Fat: 65% / Protein: 26% / Carbs: 9%

Avocado Chicken Burgers

30-MINUTE | **DAIRY-FREE** | **GLUTEN-FREE**

Possibly one of the simplest dinner recipes for the keto diet is an avocado chicken burger. Packed with healthy fats, avocado is the ultimate addition to any protein-based meal. Top these burgers with alfalfa sprouts and goat cheese or a slice of Swiss—however you serve them, they're a palate pleaser.

SERVES 4
PREP TIME: 5 MINUTES
COOK TIME: 15 MINUTES

1 pound ground chicken

½ cup almond flour

2 garlic cloves, minced

1 teaspoon onion powder

¼ teaspoon salt

⅛ teaspoon freshly ground black pepper

1 avocado, pitted, peeled, and diced

2 tablespoons olive oil

4 low-carb buns or lettuce wraps (optional)

1. In a large bowl, mix the ground chicken, almond flour, garlic, onion powder, salt, and pepper.

2. Add the avocado, gently incorporating it into the meat while forming four patties. Set aside.

3. In a large skillet, heat the olive oil over medium heat until shimmering. Add the patties to the skillet. Cook for about 8 minutes per side, or until golden brown and cooked through.

4. Serve on a low-carb bun (if using), or on its own.

TIP: If using alfalfa sprouts as a topping, it's important to note that they can sometimes carry harmful bacteria. To avoid this problem, wash them at least twice before consuming.

PER SERVING (1 PATTY): Calories: 413; Total Fat: 25.7g; Protein: 33.9g; Total Carbs: 7.9g; Fiber: 5g; Net Carbs: 2.9g
MACROS: Fat: 58% / Protein: 34% / Carbs: 8%

Stuffed Bell Peppers

DAIRY-FREE **GLUTEN-FREE** **NUT-FREE**

Bell peppers are the purses of produce—they can hold anything you'd like! This has so many flavorful ingredients, you'll want to stuff as much in as possible.

SERVES 4
PREP TIME: 10 MINUTES
COOK TIME: 45 MINUTES

4 bell peppers (any color)

8 ounces 80% lean ground beef

8 ounces ground pork

½ large yellow onion, chopped

½ tablespoon garlic powder

2 teaspoons dried basil

¾ cup canned tomato sauce or jarred sugar-free tomato sauce

½ cup shredded mozzarella cheese or nutritional yeast, plus more for serving (optional)

Chopped fresh basil, for garnishing (optional)

TIP: If you have leftover stuffing mixture, use it to top leafy greens or scramble it with eggs the next day.

TIP: To get the traditional texture of rice in the stuffed peppers, add cauliflower rice or broccoli to the skillet when you brown the meat.

1. Preheat the oven to 350°F.

2. Chop off the tops of the bell peppers and remove the seeds and ribs.

3. Set a shallow skillet over medium-high heat. Once hot, add the beef and pork plus the onion, garlic powder, and dried basil. Cook for 3 to 5 minutes, or until the meat is browned.

4. Add the tomato sauce and cheese (if using) and stir until combined.

5. Fill the cavity of each bell pepper with the mixture, then place the stuffed peppers in a baking dish. Cover with aluminum foil and bake for about 30 minutes.

6. Remove the foil and bake for another 10 minutes, or until the peppers are slightly charred and the filling is crisp.

7. Transfer the stuffed peppers to plates and sprinkle with basil (if using). Top with more cheese or nutritional yeast.

PER SERVING (¼ RECIPE): Calories: 378; Total Fat: 26g; Protein: 22g; Total Carbs: 14g; Fiber: 3g; Net Carbs: 11g
MACROS: Fat: 62% / Protein: 23% / Carbs: 15%

Chicken Fajitas

30-MINUTE **DAIRY-FREE** **NUT-FREE**

When you make fajitas at home, you can rest easy knowing that the ingredients are keto-approved. If your local Mexican restaurant includes a bit of sweetness in their spice mix, the cinnamon in this recipe will mimic that flavor (and it's also known to regulate blood sugar).

SERVES 4
PREP TIME: 10 MINUTES
COOK TIME: 20 MINUTES

1 pound boneless, skinless chicken thighs or breasts, cut into thin strips

3½ teaspoons Taco Seasoning (page 183)

1 teaspoon salt

½ teaspoon freshly ground black pepper

½ teaspoon red pepper flakes

¼ teaspoon ground cinnamon

2 tablespoons avocado oil or melted butter, divided

½ medium white onion, sliced

½ red bell pepper, cut into strips

½ green bell pepper, cut into strips

2 tablespoons Basic Broth, Chicken Variation (page 180) or store-bought chicken broth (optional)

2 to 4 low-carb tortillas, grain-free chips, or romaine lettuce leaves

1 cup shredded romaine lettuce

Sugar-free salsa, Guacamole (page 184), sour cream, and shredded cheese, for serving (optional)

1. In a large bowl, combine the chicken with the taco seasoning, salt, pepper, red pepper flakes, cinnamon, and 1 tablespoon of oil.

2. In a large, shallow skillet, heat the remaining 1 tablespoon of oil over medium-high heat. Add the onion and cook for 3 to 5 minutes, stirring occasionally, until translucent.

3. Add the red and green bell peppers and continue to cook, stirring, for another 5 minutes, until tender.

4. Add the chicken mixture and continue to cook and stir for another 2 to 3 minutes, then reduce the heat to medium, cover, and cook for about 5 minutes, or until the chicken is cooked through and no longer pink. If the chicken starts to burn, add the chicken broth (if using).

5. Remove the chicken mixture from the heat.

CONTINUED >>

6. Divide the wraps or chips among plates, sprinkle the shredded romaine on top, and spoon the chicken fajita mixture on top of the lettuce. Serve the fajitas with salsa, guacamole, sour cream, and cheese (if using).

TIP: You can buy frozen bags of sliced bell peppers and onions so you don't have to go through the task of slicing them up yourself. When shopping for low-carb tortillas, try Mission or La Tortilla Factory brands.

PER SERVING (¼ RECIPE): Calories: 216; Total Fat: 10g; Protein: 26g; Total Carbs: 4g; Fiber: 1g; Net Carbs: 3g
MACROS: Fat: 42% / Protein: 52% / Carbs: 6%

Turkey Taco Bowl

5-INGREDIENT **30-MINUTE** **ONE PAN** **DAIRY-FREE** **GLUTEN-FREE** **NUT-FREE**

Taco bowls are the perfect vessel for mixing and matching ingredients. You can swap out the ground turkey for beef or chicken, or substitute cauliflower rice for the mixed greens. Be as creative as you like and discover your favorite combination.

SERVES 1
PREP TIME: 5 MINUTES
COOK TIME: 15 MINUTES

1 tablespoon avocado oil

¼ medium red onion, diced

8 ounces 93% lean ground turkey

1 tablespoon Taco Seasoning (page 183)

2 cups chopped romaine lettuce

Guacamole (page 184), for serving

1. In a large skillet, heat the oil over medium-high heat. Add the onion and sauté for 5 to 7 minutes, until soft.

2. Add the ground turkey and cook until it's no longer pink, breaking the meat into small pieces as it cooks, about 5 minutes.

3. Add the taco seasoning and stir the mixture constantly for 1 minute. It will be crumbly.

4. Put the romaine in a bowl and top with the turkey mixture. Dollop with the guacamole and serve.

TIP: If you would like additional toppings, try adding diced tomatoes, lime wedges, black olives, or a dollop of full-fat sour cream to your bowl.

PER SERVING (ENTIRE RECIPE): Calories: 582; Total Fat: 41g; Protein: 45g; Total Carbs: 11g; Fiber: 6g; Net Carbs: 5g
MACROS: Fat: 63% / Protein: 30% / Carbs: 7%

Pecan-Stuffed Chicken Thighs

GLUTEN-FREE

If you need a fancy dish to serve guests, try these stuffed chicken thighs. The sun-dried tomatoes add both salty flavor and visual nuance to the presentation.

SERVES 4
PREP TIME: 20 MINUTES
COOK TIME: 25 MINUTES

4 ounces goat cheese

½ cup chopped pecans

2 tablespoons chopped sun-dried tomatoes

4 (5-ounce) skin-on boneless chicken thighs, butterflied

Sea salt

Freshly ground black pepper

2 tablespoons extra-virgin olive oil

¼ cup Basic Broth, Chicken Variation (page 180) or store-bought chicken broth

TIP: If you prefer, stuff the filling into butterflied pork chops instead of chicken. Just secure the edges of the chops with toothpicks to ensure that the filling doesn't ooze out.

TIP: To "butterfly" something means to slice it almost completely in half lengthwise, leaving a small bit still connected. Picture it like butterfly wings (hence the name).

1. Preheat the oven to 350°F.

2. In a small bowl, stir the goat cheese, pecans, and sun-dried tomatoes until well mixed.

3. Pat the chicken thighs dry with a paper towel. Use your fingers to loosen the skin on one thigh so it forms a pocket that's still connected at the edges.

4. Carefully spoon some goat cheese mixture into the pocket and pull the skin back to cover the filling. Repeat with the remaining thighs.

5. Season the chicken with salt and pepper.

6. In a large oven-safe skillet, heat the olive oil over medium-high heat.

7. Pan-sear the chicken, skin-side down, until crispy and golden, about 5 minutes.

8. Turn the chicken over and add the chicken broth to the skillet. Cover with a lid or aluminum foil and bake until the chicken reaches an internal temperature of 165°F, about 20 minutes. Serve hot.

PER SERVING (¼ RECIPE): Calories: 554; Total Fat: 48g; Protein: 28g Total Carbs: 3g; Fiber: 2g; Net Carbs: 1g
MACROS: Fat: 77% / Protein: 20% / Carbs: 3%

Caprese Balsamic Chicken

30-MINUTE **GLUTEN-FREE**

Whereas other vinegars are created from fermented wine, balsamic vinegar is a reduction created by boiling down grape pressings and aging them for between 12 and 100 years. Balsamic makes an excellent complement to the pesto in this recipe.

SERVES 4
PREP TIME: 10 MINUTES
COOK TIME: 20 MINUTES

3 tablespoons balsamic vinegar

1 tablespoon butter

2 (6-ounce) boneless, skinless chicken breasts, halved lengthwise

Sea salt

Freshly ground black pepper

1 tablespoon extra-virgin olive oil

¼ cup Avocado-Kale Pesto (page 188) or store-bought pesto, divided

1 tomato, cut into 4 slices

1 cup shredded mozzarella cheese

1. Preheat the oven to 400°F.

2. In a small saucepan, bring the balsamic vinegar and butter to a boil over medium heat, then reduce the heat to low and simmer until thickened, about 5 minutes. Set aside.

3. Season the chicken breasts with salt and pepper.

4. In a medium skillet, heat the olive oil over medium heat. Add the chicken and cook, turning once, until just cooked through, about 10 minutes total. Transfer the chicken to a 9-by-13-inch baking dish.

5. Spread 1 tablespoon of pesto over each piece of chicken, top each with a tomato slice, and evenly divide the cheese between the pieces.

6. Bake until the cheese is melted and golden, about 5 minutes.

7. Serve with a drizzle of the reduced balsamic vinegar.

PER SERVING (¼ RECIPE): Calories: 331; Total Fat: 22g; Protein: 27g; Total Carbs: 4g; Fiber: 1g; Net Carbs: 3g
MACROS: Fat: 60% / Protein: 34% / Carbs: 6%

Grilled Chicken Satay

DAIRY-FREE **GLUTEN-FREE**

This recipe is perfect for cookouts or dinner parties and can be served as a main dish or an appetizer. Marinate the chicken ahead of time, then grill it to perfection and serve it alongside a delicious dipping sauce.

SERVES 4
**PREP TIME: 15 MINUTES, PLUS
3 HOURS TO MARINATE**
COOK TIME: 10 MINUTES

FOR THE CHICKEN

2 pounds boneless, skinless chicken thighs, cut into 1-inch pieces

2 tablespoons coconut aminos

1 tablespoon gluten-free fish sauce (such as Red Boat brand)

1 garlic clove, minced

1 teaspoon powdered allulose

1 tablespoon freshly squeezed lime juice, plus more for serving

1 teaspoon smoked paprika

½ teaspoon ground turmeric

¼ cup chopped fresh cilantro, plus more for garnish

2 scallions, white and green parts, chopped, for garnish

FOR THE DIPPING SAUCE

½ cup full-fat coconut milk

3 tablespoons almond butter

1 tablespoon peeled, grated fresh ginger

2 garlic cloves, minced

1 tablespoon coconut aminos

1 tablespoon freshly squeezed lime juice

1 teaspoon coconut oil

½ teaspoon ground cayenne pepper

TO MAKE THE CHICKEN

1. Pat the chicken pieces dry and arrange them in a casserole dish.

2. In a medium bowl, combine the coconut aminos, fish sauce, garlic, allulose, lime juice, paprika, turmeric, and cilantro. Pour the mixture over the chicken thighs, coating them completely.

3. Cover the casserole dish with plastic wrap and refrigerate for 3 to 5 hours. In the meantime, make the dipping sauce.

4. Heat the grill or grill pan to high.

5. Thread the chicken pieces onto 12 metal skewers, dividing them evenly.

6. Grill the chicken on all sides, turning every few minutes, until it reaches an internal temperature of 165°F, about 10 minutes.

7. Garnish with lime juice, scallions, and cilantro. Serve with the dipping sauce.

TO MAKE THE DIPPING SAUCE

8. In a small saucepan over medium heat, combine the coconut milk, almond butter, ginger, garlic, coconut aminos, lime juice, coconut oil, and cayenne pepper, and stir until everything is incorporated.

9. Pour the sauce into a small bowl and serve alongside the chicken.

TIP: Want to add some spicy kick? Add 1 teaspoon of sriracha to the dipping sauce.

PER SERVING (¼ RECIPE): Calories: 425; Total Fat: 20g; Protein: 55g; Total Carbs: 6g; Fiber: 2g; Net Carbs: 4g
MACROS: Fat: 40% / Protein: 54% / Carbs: 6%

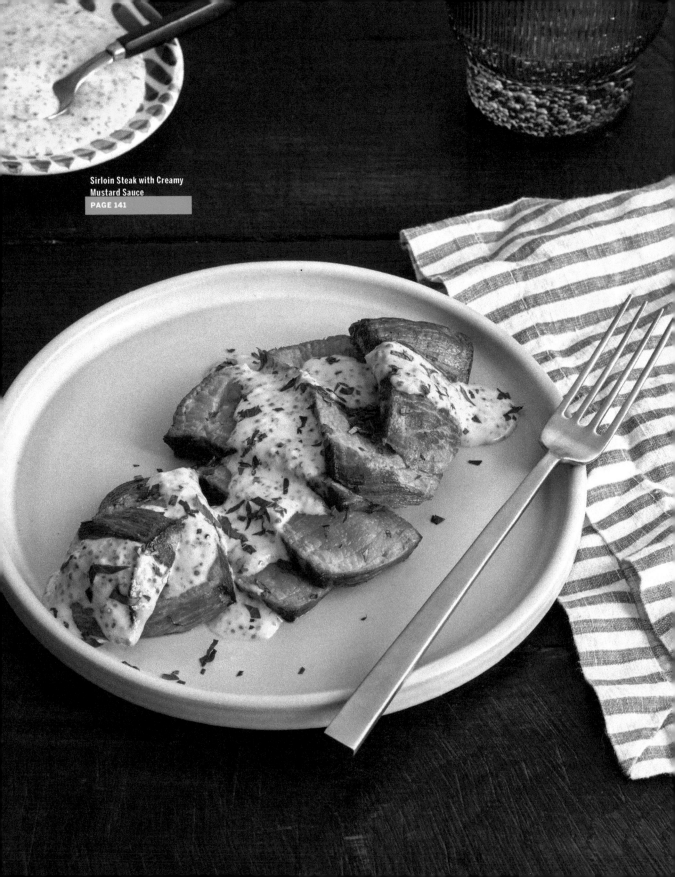

Sirloin Steak with Creamy
Mustard Sauce
PAGE 141

CHAPTER 9

Beef, Pork, and Lamb

Steak, Mushroom, and Pepper Kebabs

DAIRY-FREE GLUTEN-FREE NUT-FREE

There are endless combinations of protein and veggies you can choose from when it comes to kebabs, but these simple steak and mushroom kebabs are known crowd pleasers. Try serving them with a side of field greens and some Ranch Dressing (page 187) or a simple vinaigrette.

SERVES 4
PREP TIME: 15 MINUTES
COOK TIME: 20 MINUTES

1 pound sirloin steak, cut into large cubes

8 ounces white button mushrooms or baby bella mushrooms

1 red bell pepper, cut into 1-inch squares

1 green bell pepper, cut into 1-inch squares

3 tablespoons extra-virgin olive oil

Salt

Freshly ground black pepper

> **TIP:** Turn these kebabs into chicken fajitas. Combine 8 ounces of cubed boneless, skinless chicken breasts or thighs; season with Taco Seasoning (page 183), salt, and pepper; thread onto skewers; and cook for 10 to 14 minutes, until cooked through. Serve with lime wedges.

1. Preheat the grill or grill pan to medium-high heat.

2. In a large bowl, combine the cubed steak, mushrooms, and red and green bell peppers. Add the olive oil and season with salt and pepper. Toss to combine. Alternate pieces of steak, mushroom, and bell pepper on metal skewers.

3. Grill for 6 to 8 minutes per side, until the steak is cooked through and the veggies are charred. Alternatively, cook the kebabs in a large skillet over medium-high heat.

4. Remove from the heat, slide the steak and mushrooms from the skewers, and serve. Refrigerate leftovers in an airtight container for up to 5 days.

PER SERVING (¼ RECIPE): Calories: 340; Total Fat: 24g; Protein: 27g; Total Carbs: 5g; Fiber: 1g; Net Carbs: 4g
MACROS: Fat: 63% / Protein: 31% / Carbs: 6%

FAJITA VARIATION PER SERVING (¼ RECIPE): Calories: 416; Total Fat: 24g; Protein: 39g; Total Carbs: 9g; Fiber: 3g; Net Carbs: 6g
MACROS: Fat: 53% / Protein: 38% / Carbs: 9%

Italian Meatballs

GLUTEN-FREE

The tiny pinch of allspice in these meatballs might not seem important, but you will miss the flavor in the finished meatballs if you leave it out. Plus, it's got all kinds of health benefits. Allspice is high in vitamin C, iron, calcium, magnesium, copper, manganese, iron, and magnesium. It can reduce blood pressure, cut the risk of diabetes, and relieve symptoms associated with PMS and arthritis.

SERVES 4
PREP TIME: 20 MINUTES
COOK TIME: 20 MINUTES

12 ounces 80% lean ground beef

¾ cup grated Parmesan cheese

½ cup almond flour

¼ medium sweet onion, minced

1 large egg

1 teaspoon minced garlic

1 teaspoon dried basil

½ teaspoon dried oregano

Pinch ground allspice

2 tablespoons extra-virgin olive oil

1. Preheat the oven to 350°F. Line a baking sheet with parchment paper.

2. In a large bowl, mix the ground beef, Parmesan, almond flour, onion, egg, garlic, basil, oregano, and allspice until well blended.

3. Roll the beef mixture into 1½-inch balls.

4. In a large skillet, heat the oil over medium-high heat. Add the meatballs and brown all over for about 10 minutes, then transfer them to the prepared baking sheet.

5. Bake the meatballs until just cooked through, about 10 minutes.

6. Serve plain or with your favorite sauce.

PER SERVING (¼ RECIPE): Calories: 449; Total Fat: 36g; Protein: 24g; Total Carbs: 7g; Fiber: 2g; Net Carbs: 5g
MACROS: Fat: 71% / Protein: 23% / Carbs: 6%

Cheeseburger Meat Loaf

GLUTEN-FREE NUT-FREE

Who needs a bun when you can take all the goodness of a classic juicy cheese-burger and transform it into a delicious meat loaf? Double the recipe and you'll have plenty of leftovers for the next day. You're going to want them!

SERVES 1
PREP TIME: 10 MINUTES
COOK TIME: 45 MINUTES

6 ounces 80% lean ground beef

¼ cup shredded cheddar cheese

1 large egg, beaten

¼ medium white onion, diced

1 teaspoon salt

1 teaspoon garlic powder

2 tablespoons tomato paste

1 tablespoon yellow mustard

1 tablespoon coconut aminos

1. Preheat the oven to 350°F. Line a baking sheet with parchment paper.

2. In a large bowl, combine the ground beef, cheese, egg, onion, salt, and garlic powder.

3. Using your hands, gently mix the ingredients just enough to combine them. (Overmixing can make the meat loaf tough.)

4. Transfer the mixture to the prepared baking sheet and form it into a loaf shape. Bake for 30 minutes.

5. Meanwhile, in a small bowl, whisk the tomato paste, mustard, and coconut aminos until fully combined.

6. Remove the meat loaf from the oven and spread the sauce mixture evenly over the top.

7. Return to the oven and bake for another 15 minutes, or until cooked through and browned on top.

PER SERVING (ENTIRE RECIPE): Calories: 737; Total Fat: 57g; Protein: 42g; Total Carbs: 14g; Fiber: 4g; Net Carbs: 10g
MACROS: Fat: 70% / Protein: 23% / Carbs: 7%

Sirloin Steak with Creamy Mustard Sauce

30-MINUTE | GLUTEN-FREE | NUT-FREE

Who has the time to cook restaurant-quality meals every night? Well, with this recipe, you do. The creamy mustard sauce makes this dish—no exaggeration—Michelin star–worthy. Just make sure you use a robust mustard in the sauce (not the bright yellow stuff).

SERVES 4
PREP TIME: 10 MINUTES
COOK TIME: 15 MINUTES

4 (4-ounce) sirloin steaks, at room temperature

2 tablespoons extra-virgin olive oil

Sea salt

Freshly ground black pepper

1 cup heavy (whipping) cream

¼ cup grainy mustard

1 teaspoon chopped, fresh thyme

1. Preheat the oven to broil.

2. Rub the steaks all over with the olive oil, then season with salt and pepper.

3. Place the steaks on a baking sheet and broil for 7 minutes per side for medium rare.

4. While the steaks are broiling, place a small saucepan over medium heat and pour in the heavy cream and mustard. Bring the sauce to a boil, then reduce the heat to low and simmer until very thick, 5 to 6 minutes. Remove from the heat and stir in the thyme.

5. Let the steaks rest for 10 minutes before serving them topped with the mustard sauce.

TIP: Double the sauce and save the extra in a sealed container in the refrigerator for up to 5 days. Reheat it in a skillet and pour over fish, poultry, pork, or roasted vegetables for a real treat.

PER SERVING (¼ RECIPE): Calories: 505; Total Fat: 43g; Protein: 24g; Total Carbs: 2g; Fiber: 0g; Net Carbs: 2g
MACROS: Fat: 78% / Protein: 21% / Carbs: 1%

Casserole au Gratin

GLUTEN-FREE

Cream cheese is the secret ingredient for a decadent, smooth sauce. You will be using only about ½ cup of cream cheese, so use the rest in other recipes because it will only keep for about a week after being opened. Cream cheese is lovely in omelets, baking, pâté, meatballs, sauces, and ice cream.

SERVES 4
PREP TIME: 25 MINUTES
COOK TIME: 30 MINUTES

4 tablespoons butter, melted, plus more for greasing

5 cups small cauliflower florets

2 cups diced lean ham

4 ounces full-fat cream cheese, at room temperature

½ cup whole milk, plain Greek yogurt

1 jalapeño pepper, seeded and diced

1 scallion, white and green parts, chopped

1 cup almond flour

1 teaspoon chopped fresh parsley

1. Preheat the oven to 350°F.

2. Lightly butter an 8-inch casserole dish.

3. Place a large saucepan filled with water over high heat and bring the water to a boil. Add the cauliflower and boil until tender-crisp, about 4 minutes. Drain and transfer to a large bowl. Add the ham to the bowl and toss to combine.

4. In a small bowl, whisk together the cream cheese, yogurt, jalapeño, and scallion until well mixed.

5. Stir the cream cheese mixture into the cauliflower mixture, being sure to coat the vegetables and ham. Spoon the mixture into the casserole dish.

6. In a small bowl, stir together the almond flour, melted butter, and parsley until the mixture looks like coarse crumbs. Sprinkle the topping evenly over the casserole.

7. Bake until the topping is lightly browned and all the mixture is bubbly, about 20 minutes. Serve.

PER SERVING (¼ RECIPE): Calories: 501; Total Fat: 38g; Protein: 20g; Total Carbs: 14g; Fiber: 7g; Net Carbs: 7g
MACROS: Fat: 70% / Protein: 18% / Carbs: 12%

Walnut-Crusted Pork Chops

5-INGREDIENT | **30-MINUTE** | **GLUTEN-FREE**

Pork chops are inexpensive, and with the right ketogenic "breading" (in this case, crushed walnuts and grated Parmesan cheese), you can take the flavor anywhere you want. Thick-cut pork chops work best because they stay juicy throughout the cooking process. Serve this over zoodles for a great meal.

SERVES 2
PREP TIME: 10 MINUTES
COOK TIME: 20 MINUTES

3 tablespoons crushed walnuts

3 tablespoons grated
   Parmesan cheese

Pinch sea salt

Pinch freshly ground
   black pepper

1 large egg

2 (8-ounce) boneless pork chops

1. Preheat the oven to 400°F. Line a rimmed baking sheet with parchment paper.

2. In a shallow dish, mix the walnuts, Parmesan, salt, and pepper.

3. In another shallow dish, lightly beat the egg.

4. One at a time, dip each pork chop in the egg, coat it with the walnut-and-Parmesan mixture, and place it on the baking sheet.

5. Bake the chops for 10 minutes, flip them, and continue baking until they reach 145°F in the center, about 10 minutes more. Serve immediately.

PER SERVING (½ RECIPE): Calories: 352; Total Fat: 17g; Protein: 47g; Total Carbs: 2g; Fiber: 1g; Net Carbs: 1g
MACROS: Fat: 43% / Protein: 53% / Carbs: 4%

Pan-Grilled Lamb Chops with Pesto

5-INGREDIENT **30-MINUTE** **ONE PAN** **DAIRY-FREE** **GLUTEN-FREE**

When shopping for lamb, look for firm, pink flesh with white fat marbling, not yellow. Organic, grass-fed meat contains more omega-3 fatty acids because these levels are dependent on what the animal eats. Even "regular" lamb is very high in vitamin B_{12}, protein, selenium, and vitamin B_3. Eating lamb can reduce your risk of heart disease and can help regulate blood sugar.

SERVES 4
PREP TIME: 5 MINUTES, PLUS 15 MINUTES TO REACH ROOM TEMPERATURE
COOK TIME: 10 MINUTES

4 (4-ounce) lamb chops

Sea salt

Freshly ground black pepper

2 tablespoons extra-virgin olive oil

¼ cup Avocado-Kale Pesto (page 188) or store-bought pesto, divided

1. Season the lamb chops with salt and pepper.

2. Let the lamb chops sit, covered, until they reach room temperature, 15 to 20 minutes.

3. In a large skillet, heat the olive oil over medium-high heat.

4. Sear the chops in the skillet for about 5 minutes per side for medium rare.

5. Let the lamb chops rest for 10 minutes before serving them with 1 tablespoon of pesto per chop.

PER SERVING (¼ RECIPE): Calories: 413; Total Fat: 32g; Protein: 32g Total Carbs: 2g; Fiber: 2g; Net Carbs: 0g
MACROS: Fat: 70% / Protein: 30% / Carbs: 0%

Beef and Broccoli

30-MINUTE **ONE PAN** **DAIRY-FREE** **GLUTEN-FREE** **NUT-FREE**

Skip the Chinese takeout and make an upgraded keto version of this popular dish. Serve it on its own or with cauliflower rice for an indulgent yet guilt-free meal.

SERVES 1
PREP TIME: 10 MINUTES
COOK TIME: 20 MINUTES

1 tablespoon coconut oil

6 ounces skirt steak, cut into thin, 2-inch strips

2 garlic cloves, minced

½ teaspoon minced fresh ginger

1½ cups broccoli florets

¼ cup water

¼ cup coconut aminos

Juice of ½ lemon

½ teaspoon apple cider vinegar

Pinch red pepper flakes (optional)

Salt

Freshly ground black pepper

1. In a large skillet, melt the coconut oil over medium-high heat. Add the steak and sauté for 5 to 7 minutes until cooked through. Transfer to a plate.

2. Lower the heat to medium and add the garlic and ginger. Cook and stir for about 1 minute, until fragrant. Add the broccoli and cook for 2 minutes, until lightly browned.

3. Add the water, cover, and reduce the heat to medium-low. Cook for 10 minutes, stirring occasionally, until the broccoli is tender.

4. Add the coconut aminos, lemon juice, vinegar, red pepper flakes (if using), and the reserved steak to the broccoli. Sauté, tossing to combine, for 1 to 2 minutes until warmed through.

5. Season with salt and pepper to taste. Serve.

PER SERVING (ENTIRE RECIPE): Calories: 458; Total Fat: 26g; Protein: 35g; Total Carbs: 21g; Fiber: 4g; Net Carbs: 17g
MACROS: Fat: 51% / Protein: 31% / Carbs: 18%

Pork Fried Rice

30-MINUTE | **GLUTEN-FREE** | **NUT-FREE**

This dish is a fan favorite that will not disappoint—whether you are eating keto or not. Your non-keto friends might even be shocked when you make this for them and they realize the "rice" is actually cauliflower.

SERVES 1
PREP TIME: 10 MINUTES
COOK TIME: 15 MINUTES

½ head cauliflower, cut into small florets

1 tablespoon avocado oil

1 (6-ounce) pork tenderloin, cut into thin strips

1 tablespoon butter or ghee

1 scallion, white and green parts, finely sliced and divided

1 teaspoon minced fresh ginger

1 garlic clove, minced

1 large egg, beaten

1 tablespoon coconut aminos

1 teaspoon toasted sesame oil

1. In a food processor, process the cauliflower florets until the mixture resembles rice.

2. In a large skillet, heat the oil over medium heat. Add the pork strips and sauté for 4 to 5 minutes, until golden on both sides, then transfer to a plate and set aside.

3. In the same skillet, combine the butter, cauliflower "rice," and the white parts of the scallion. Cook for about 5 minutes, or until the cauliflower begins to soften slightly.

4. Add the ginger and garlic and stir for about 30 seconds. Add the beaten egg and cook, stirring continuously, until scrambled. Add the pork and coconut aminos and cook for another 2 minutes, stirring continuously, until well combined.

5. Remove from the heat and stir in the sesame oil and green parts of the scallion. Serve.

PER SERVING (ENTIRE RECIPE): Calories: 565; Total Fat: 41g; Protein: 39g; Total Carbs: 10g; Fiber: 4g; Net Carbs: 6g
MACROS: Fat: 65% / Protein: 28% / Carbs: 7%

Steak and Egg Bibimbap

30-MINUTE **GLUTEN-FREE** **NUT-FREE**

Bibimbap means "mixed rice" in Korean. Although this recipe is unlike a traditional version, it has the key ingredients: beef, a runny egg, and vegetables. It's a great dish to make when you have leftover veggies in the refrigerator, because you can throw in just about anything. You can also make this recipe with ground turkey or beef instead of steak.

SERVES 2
PREP TIME: 10 MINUTES
COOK TIME: 15 MINUTES

FOR THE STEAK

8 ounces skirt steak

Salt

Freshly ground black pepper

1 tablespoon butter or ghee

FOR THE EGG AND CAULIFLOWER "RICE"

2 tablespoons butter or ghee, divided

2 large eggs

1 large cucumber, peeled and cut into matchsticks

1 tablespoon coconut aminos or gluten-free soy sauce

1 cup riced cauliflower

Salt

Freshly ground black pepper

TO MAKE THE STEAK

1. Pat the steak dry and season both sides with salt and pepper.

2. In a large skillet, melt the butter over high heat. Add the steak and sear for about 3 minutes on each side for medium rare.

3. Transfer to a cutting board and let rest for at least 5 minutes. Slice the steak across the grain and divide it between two bowls.

TO MAKE THE EGG AND CAULIFLOWER "RICE"

4. In the same skillet, melt 1 tablespoon of butter over medium-high heat. When the butter is very hot, crack the eggs into it. When the whites have cooked through, after 2 to 3 minutes, carefully transfer the eggs to a plate. Turn off the heat and let the skillet cool.

5. In a small bowl, combine the cucumber and coconut aminos and set aside to marinate.

CONTINUED >>

6. Wipe out the skillet and place it back over medium-high heat. Melt the remaining 1 tablespoon of butter and add the cauliflower, season with salt and pepper, and stir, cooking for 5 minutes until softened. Turn the heat up to high at the end of the cooking to get a nice crisp on the cauliflower.

7. Divide the cauliflower between two bowls.

8. Top the "rice" in each bowl with an egg, the steak, and the marinated cucumber matchsticks. Serve.

TIP: You can add so many vegetables and other ingredients to a bibimbap, so take a look in your refrigerator and get creative. Delicious add-ins or toppings include kimchi, sriracha, bean sprouts, carrot matchsticks, chopped mushrooms, and chopped scallions.

PER SERVING (½ RECIPE): Calories: 523; Total Fat: 43g; Protein: 29g; Total Carbs: 7g; Fiber: 2g; Net Carbs: 5g
MACROS: Fat: 73% / Protein: 22% / Carbs: 5%

Sloppy Joe Casserole

GLUTEN-FREE   NUT-FREE

Sloppy joes are a classic comfort food—cheap and easy to make at home on a budget. This low-carb sloppy joe casserole takes all those nostalgic flavors and brings them together in a much healthier way. You won't miss the buns for a second when you dive into this delicious beefy casserole. Using riced cauliflower is a great way to add volume to a recipe while keeping the calories and carbs low. If you like your sloppy joes spicy, add sliced jalapeños on top for an extra kick. A dollop of sour cream is also a nice addition. You can substitute ground chicken, turkey, or bison for a leaner, lower-calorie version.

SERVES 4
PREP TIME: 10 MINUTES
COOK TIME: 30 MINUTES

½ cup heavy (whipping) cream

4 ounces full-fat cream cheese

1 cup shredded cheddar cheese, divided

2 cups riced cauliflower

Salt

Freshly ground black pepper

1 tablespoon butter

½ cup diced white onion

1 pound 80% lean ground beef (see tip)

½ cup sugar-free ketchup

1 tablespoon Worcestershire sauce

1 tablespoon smoked paprika

1. Preheat the oven to 400°F.

2. In a medium, microwave-safe bowl, combine the heavy cream and cream cheese. Microwave for 30 seconds, then whisk until the cream cheese is completely melted.

3. Add ½ cup of cheddar cheese and the cauliflower. Season with salt and pepper and fold to combine. Pour the mixture into an 8-by-8-inch casserole dish. Set aside.

4. In a medium skillet, melt the butter over medium-high heat. When it foams, add the onion and cook for 2 minutes, until soft. Add the beef, using a spatula to break it into bite-size pieces, for 5 minutes, until cooked through.

CONTINUED >>

5. Drain the pan of most of the excess liquid, then add the ketchup, Worcestershire sauce, smoked paprika, and more salt and pepper to taste.

6. Pour the sloppy joe mixture over the cauliflower mixture, then top with the remaining ½ cup of cheddar cheese. Bake for 15 to 20 minutes, until hot and bubbling.

7. Let the casserole cool for 5 minutes before serving.

TIP: Look for lean ground beef with 20 percent fat or less. Buying fatty ground beef makes the dish greasy. Plus, it means you're paying for fat, not meat. It's worth the extra cost to purchase extra-lean ground beef (7 percent fat) when you can, because the quality of the finished recipe will be noticeable.

PER SERVING (¼ RECIPE): Calories: 667; Total Fat: 56g; Protein: 31g; Total Carbs: 11g; Fiber: 3g; Net Carbs: 8g
MACROS: Fat: 75% / Protein: 19% / Carbs: 6%

Lasagna Dip

30-MINUTE **GLUTEN-FREE** **NUT-FREE**

Scoop up this lasagna dip using pork rinds, red bell peppers, zucchini, or even cheese crisps. You can make it in 30 minutes, but if you prefer, prep the recipe ahead of time and bake it just before you're ready to serve. Substitute ground chicken, ground turkey, or Italian sausage to put your own twist on the dish.

SERVES 4
PREP TIME: 10 MINUTES
COOK TIME: 20 MINUTES

1 pound 80% lean ground beef

2 large eggs

1 cup whole milk ricotta

¼ cup grated Parmesan cheese

1 tablespoon Italian seasoning, divided

1 cup no-sugar-added marinara sauce, divided

1 cup shredded mozzarella cheese, divided

TIP: You can also add a layer of riced cauliflower to the bottom of this dish to bulk it up and turn it into a full meal.

PER SERVING (¼ RECIPE): Calories: 557; Total Fat: 41g; Protein: 38g; Total Carbs: 7g; Fiber: 1g; Net Carbs: 6g
MACROS: Fat: 66% / Protein: 29% / Carbs: 5%

1. Preheat the oven to 400°F.

2. Set a large, oven-safe skillet over medium-high heat. Once hot, put in the ground beef. Cook for 5 minutes, using a wooden spoon or spatula to break up the meat into bite-size pieces, until browned and cooked through. Scoop the meat onto a plate lined with paper towels. Drain any excess grease from the skillet.

3. In a medium bowl, whisk together the eggs, ricotta, Parmesan cheese, and 2 teaspoons of Italian seasoning.

4. In the skillet, layer ½ cup of ricotta mixture followed by half the ground beef, ½ cup of marinara sauce, and ½ cup of mozzarella. Repeat the layers, then top with the remaining 1 teaspoon of Italian seasoning.

5. Bake for 15 minutes, until the cheese on top is melted and golden.

6. Let rest for 10 minutes before serving.

7. Freeze leftovers for up to 6 months.

Cubano Pork Chops

30-MINUTE **GLUTEN-FREE** **NUT-FREE**

This recipe is the iconic Cubano pressed sandwich reimagined as a knife and fork entrée. The combination of thinly sliced ham, Swiss cheese, dill pickle, and yellow mustard works perfectly. Cubano pork chops are great served with sautéed veggies and riced cauliflower.

SERVES 4
PREP TIME: 10 MINUTES
COOK TIME: 15 MINUTES

2 pounds boneless pork loin, cut into 1-inch-thick chops

Salt

Freshly ground black pepper

1 tablespoon avocado oil

2 tablespoons yellow mustard

½ cup sliced dill pickles

8 ounces sliced ham

4 slices Swiss cheese

1. Preheat the oven to 450°F.

2. Season the pork liberally with salt and pepper.

3. In a large, oven-safe skillet, heat the oil over medium-high heat until shimmering. Add the pork and sear for about 3 minutes per side, until golden.

4. Brush a thin coat of mustard over each pork chop. Layer with dill pickles, ham, and Swiss cheese.

5. Bake the pork chops for 5 minutes, until the cheese has melted. Let rest for 5 minutes before serving.

TIP: Buying an entire pork loin is a great way to save money on meal prep. You can cut the pork loin into 1-inch chops and freeze them individually, and use the end cuts for Barbecue Pork Bites (page 153). Frozen pork loin thaws quickly and can be grilled or pan-seared for an easy weeknight meal.

PER SERVING (¼ RECIPE): Calories: 578; Total Fat: 32g; Protein: 66g; Total Carbs: 3g; Fiber: 1g; Net Carbs: 2g
MACROS: Fat: 50%; Protein: 48%; Carbs: 2%

Barbecue Pork Bites

DAIRY-FREE GLUTEN-FREE NUT-FREE

These pork bites are a great weeknight recipe when you're in the mood for barbecue but don't have eight hours to slow-cook a pork shoulder. Dip the bites in Ranch Dressing (page 187) or make them ahead along with riced cauliflower for part of your weekly meal prep. You can also make this recipe using cubed chicken breast for a change of pace or if you don't eat pork.

SERVES 4
PREP TIME: 10 MINUTES, PLUS
30 MINUTES TO MARINATE
COOK TIME: 15 MINUTES

2 pounds pork tenderloin, cut into 1½-inch pieces

2 tablespoons avocado oil, divided

1 tablespoon barbecue spice rub

¼ cup sugar-free barbecue sauce

¼ cup thinly sliced scallions, green part only

½ cup Ranch Dressing (page 187) or store-bought ranch dressing, for serving

1. In a large bowl, toss the pork with 1 tablespoon of avocado oil and the barbecue spice rub. Make sure the pork is coated on all sides. Cover and marinate for 30 minutes in the refrigerator.

2. In a large skillet, heat the remaining 1 tablespoon of avocado oil over medium-high heat until shimmering. Add the pork, making sure not to crowd the pan. Cook for 5 to 7 minutes on each side, stirring occasionally, until the pork has a golden crust on all sides and reaches an internal temperature of 155°F. Remove from the heat.

3. Add the barbecue sauce to the pork bites and toss to coat them well. Garnish with the scallions and serve with the ranch dressing for dipping.

TIP: Change up the seasoning so you don't get bored eating the same flavor pork bites every time. Cajun seasoning, Caribbean jerk seasoning, or just salt and pepper are all tasty variations of this recipe.

PER SERVING (¼ RECIPE): Calories: 465; Total Fat: 28g; Protein: 47g; Total Carbs: 3g; Fiber: 0g; Net Carbs: 3g
MACROS: Fat: 54% / Protein: 43% / Carbs: 3%

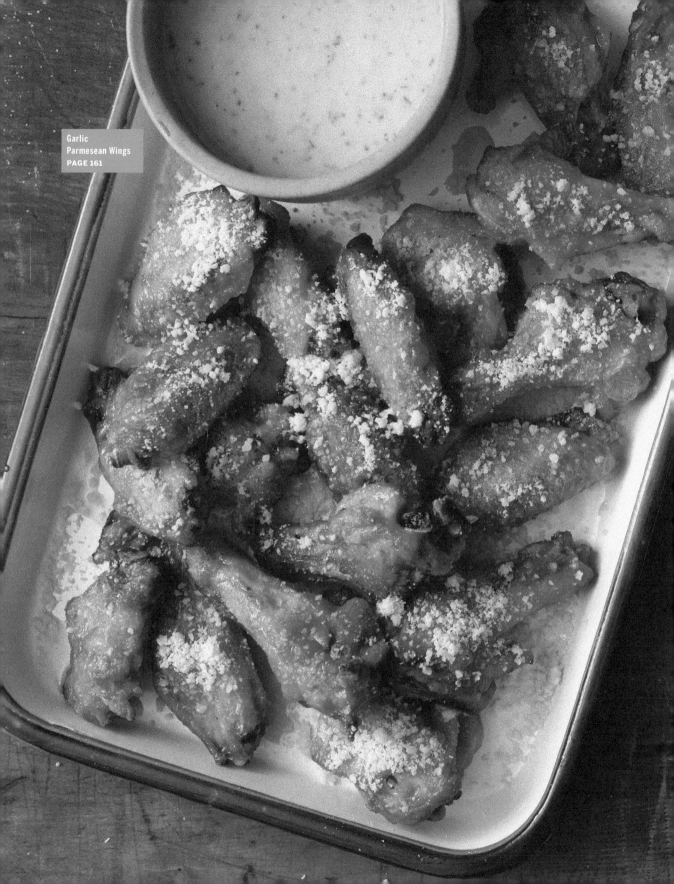

Garlic
Parmesean Wings
PAGE 161

CHAPTER 10

Apps and Snacks

Parmesan Pepperoni Chips

5-INGREDIENT | 30-MINUTE | ONE PAN | GLUTEN-FREE | NUT-FREE

If you're a "chip and dipper" at heart, one of the things you may be missing on a keto diet are chips. Enter: Parmesan pepperoni chips. They'll satisfy that craving for a crispy snack! Reheat leftovers in the oven to bring back their crispness.

MAKES ABOUT 84 CHIPS
PREP TIME: 5 MINUTES
COOK TIME: 15 MINUTES

1 (6-ounce) bag sliced pepperoni

½ cup finely grated
  Parmesan cheese

1. Preheat the oven to 425°F. Line a baking sheet with parchment paper.

2. Lay the pepperoni slices on the prepared baking sheet in a single layer.

3. Bake for 10 minutes, then remove from the oven and blot with a paper towel to soak up the grease.

4. Lightly cover the pepperoni with the Parmesan and return to the oven. Bake for another 3 to 4 minutes, until the pepperoni slices look crispy.

5. Remove from the oven and transfer the pepperoni to paper towels to absorb any remaining grease. Serve.

TIP: These little chips are great for dipping in Ranch Dressing (page 187), blue cheese dressing, or Guacamole (page 184). Just be sure to add the additional carbs to your total.

PER SERVING (ABOUT 14 CHIPS): Calories 174; Total Fat: 15g; Protein: 10g; Total Carbs: 0g; Fiber: 0g; Net Carbs: 0g
MACROS: Fat: 77% / Protein: 23% / Carbs: 0%

Seedy Crackers

DAIRY-FREE **GLUTEN-FREE** **VEGETARIAN**

These grain-free crackers satisfy a craving for something crunchy without compromising your keto diet. Enjoy them topped with smoked salmon or a slice of avocado sprinkled with salt.

SERVES 4
PREP TIME: 25 MINUTES
COOK TIME: 15 MINUTES

1 cup almond flour

1 tablespoon sesame seeds

1 tablespoon flaxseed

1 tablespoon chia seeds

¼ teaspoon baking soda

¼ teaspoon salt

Freshly ground black pepper

1 large egg, at room
   temperature, beaten

1. Preheat the oven to 350°F.

2. In a large bowl, combine the almond flour, sesame seeds, flaxseed, chia seeds, baking soda, salt, and pepper, and stir well. Add the beaten egg and stir again to form the dough into a ball.

3. Place the dough on a piece of parchment paper. Cover with a second layer of parchment and, using a rolling pin, roll the dough to an ⅛-inch thickness, aiming for a rectangular shape.

4. Using a cookie cutter, cut the dough into 1- to 2-inch circles. Remove the excess dough and transfer the circles with their parchment to a baking sheet. (You can reshape any leftover dough into additional circles, if needed.)

5. Bake until crispy and slightly golden, 10 to 15 minutes, depending on thickness. Alternatively, you can bake the rolled dough prior to cutting break it into free-form crackers.

6. Cool on a wire rack for 10 minutes. Serve.

PER SERVING (6 CRACKERS): Calories: 119, Total Fat: 9g; Protein: 5g; Total Carbs: 4g, Fiber: 3g; Net Carbs: 1g
MACROS: Fat: 68% / Protein: 17% / Carbs: 15%

Pumpkin Pecan Fat Bombs

GLUTEN-FREE VEGETARIAN

These tasty nuggets are like tiny pumpkin cheesecakes: warmly spiced and slightly nutty. The combination of tart goat cheese, rich pumpkin, and buttery pecans is addictive, so double the batch to store some in the freezer for later. You can swap sweet potato for pumpkin (or almonds for pecans) without significantly changing the macros.

MAKES 12 FAT BOMBS
PREP TIME: 10 MINUTES, PLUS 30 MINUTES TO CHILL

½ cup butter, at room temperature

½ cup goat cheese, at room temperature

1 teaspoon erythritol

¼ teaspoon ground cinnamon

¼ teaspoon ground nutmeg

½ cup pure pumpkin puree

¼ cup finely chopped pecans

1. In a medium bowl, stir together the butter, goat cheese, erythritol, cinnamon, and nutmeg until very smooth.

2. Stir in the pumpkin puree and pecans until well blended.

3. Put the mixture in the refrigerator until it is firm enough to roll into balls, about 30 minutes.

4. Use a tablespoon to scoop out the fat-bomb and roll it into balls. Place the balls in the freezer in an 8-by-8-inch baking dish until very firm.

5. Serve immediately or transfer to a container with a lid and store in the freezer for up to 1 month.

TIP: Be sure to buy pure pumpkin puree for this recipe, not pumpkin pie filling, which is full of sugar.

PER SERVING (1 FAT BOMB): Calories: 100; Total Fat: 10g; Protein: 1g; Total Carbs: 1g; Fiber: 1g; Net Carbs: 0g
MACROS: Fat: 90% / Protein: 4% / Carbs: 6%

Jalapeño Poppers

5-INGREDIENT **GLUTEN-FREE** **NUT-FREE**

Spicy, cheesy, and crunchy, jalapeño poppers hit the spot. The poppers you find at restaurants are deep fried, but these are wrapped in bacon and baked. The mess is nonexistent, and the crunch and flavor are spot on. Make these poppers in bulk for feeding a crowd.

SERVES 4
PREP TIME: 15 MINUTES
COOK TIME: 20 MINUTES

4 ounces full-fat cream cheese, at room temperature

⅓ cup shredded cheddar cheese

4 jalapeño peppers, halved and seeded

4 slices bacon, halved widthwise

2 tablespoons sour cream

1. Preheat the oven to 375°F. Line a baking sheet with parchment paper.

2. In a small bowl, mix together the cream cheese and cheddar cheese until well combined. Spoon the cheese mixture evenly into each jalapeño half.

3. Wrap each jalapeño half with a piece of bacon and secure with a toothpick. Place on the prepared baking sheet.

4. Bake for 15 to 20 minutes or until the bacon is crisp.

5. Top each pepper half with sour cream. Serve immediately.

TIP: Wear gloves when handling the peppers or wash your hands thoroughly afterward. Don't touch your eyes after touching a jalapeño pepper with bare hands.

PER SERVING (2 PEPPER HALVES): Calories: 189; Total Fat: 17g; Protein: 7g; Total Carbs: 3g; Fiber: <1g; Net Carbs: 3g
MACROS: Fat: 78% / Protein: 15% / Carbs: 7%

Smoked Salmon Crudités

30-MINUTE | **ONE BOWL** | **DAIRY-FREE** | **GLUTEN-FREE** | **NUT-FREE**

Full of heart-healthy omega-3 fatty acids, this light dip is perfect served with fresh veggies such as the endive and cucumbers in this recipe, atop Seedy Crackers (page 157), or even as a light lunch with a fresh green salad. You can make extra at the beginning of the week to have as a quick snack or grab-and-go lunch. For the highest amount of omega-3s, always look for wild-caught salmon as opposed to farm-raised salmon.

MAKES 4
PREP TIME: 10 MINUTES

6 ounces smoked, wild salmon, roughly chopped

2 tablespoons Keto Mayonnaise (page 186) or store-bought mayonnaise

1 tablespoon Dijon mustard

1 tablespoon chopped scallions, green part only

2 teaspoons chopped capers

½ teaspoon dried dill

4 endive spears or hearts of romaine

½ English cucumber, cut into ¼-inch-thick rounds

1. In a small bowl, combine the salmon, mayonnaise, mustard, scallions, capers, and dill. Mix well.

2. Top the endive spears and cucumber rounds with a spoonful of smoked salmon mixture and serve chilled.

TIP: You can substitute canned salmon (removing bones and skin), chipped sardines, or mackerel for the smoked salmon, if you prefer.

PER SERVING (1 CRUDITÉ): Calories: 106; Total Fat: 7g; Protein: 8g; Total Carbs: 2g; Fiber: 1g; Net Carbs: 1g
MACROS: Fat: 62% / Protein: 33% / Carbs: 5%

Garlic Parmesan Wings

5-INGREDIENT | **GLUTEN-FREE** | **NUT-FREE**

Bone-in, garlic-Parmesan wings from Wingstop are legendary, and thankfully, they are also keto-friendly. Here's a super easy, at-home version. To recreate the whole wing takeout experience, serve them with celery sticks and blue cheese or Ranch Dressing (page 187).

SERVES 5
PREP TIME: 5 MINUTES
COOK TIME: 1 HOUR

2½ pounds party chicken wing pieces (20 to 22 wings), patted dry

8 tablespoons (1 stick) butter, melted

1 tablespoon garlic salt or 1 tablespoon minced garlic

½ cup grated Parmesan cheese

1. Preheat the oven to 375°F. Line a rimmed baking sheet with parchment paper.

2. Place the chicken wings on the prepared baking sheet. Bake for 1 hour, flipping the wings halfway through, then transfer to a bowl.

3. Add the butter and garlic salt and toss gently to coat. Top with the Parmesan and serve.

> **TIP:** You can give these some spice with sriracha sauce or hot sauce. Just be sure to add the additional carbs to your total.

PER SERVING (4 CHICKEN WINGS): Calories: 469; Total Fat: 40g; Protein: 26g; Total Carbs: 1g; Fiber: 0g; Net Carbs: 1g
MACROS: Fat: 77% / Protein: 22% / Carbs: 1%

Blackberry "Cheesecake" Bites

DAIRY-FREE **GLUTEN-FREE** **VEGETARIAN**

That famous cheesecake restaurant doesn't have a thing on this snack. These satisfying bites are so much healthier with the fat from the coconut, protein from the almonds, and antioxidants from the blackberries—not to mention the sugar-free sweetness. It's a one-two-three-four power punch. Who says cheesecake isn't good for you?

SERVES 4
PREP TIME: 5 MINUTES, PLUS OVERNIGHT TO SOAK AND 1 HOUR, 30 MINUTES TO SET

1½ cups almonds, soaked overnight

1 cup fresh blackberries

⅓ cup coconut oil, melted

⅓ cup powdered allulose

¼ cup full-fat coconut cream

¼ cup freshly squeezed lemon juice

1. Line a 12-cup muffin tin with cupcake liners.

2. In a blender, combine the soaked almonds, blackberries, coconut oil, allulose, coconut cream, and lemon juice. Blend on high until the mixture is whipped and fluffy.

3. Divide the mixture equally among the muffin cups.

4. Place the muffin tin in the freezer for 1 hour and 30 minutes to allow the cheesecake bites to set. Serve cold.

TIP: This dessert works great prepared in advance because you can keep it in the freezer. To thaw, place the bites on the countertop for 1 hour to come to room temperature.

PER SERVING (3 BITES): Calories: 534; Total Fat: 50g; Protein: 12g; Total Carbs: 17g; Fiber: 9g; Net Carbs: 8g
MACROS: Fat: 79% / Protein: 8% / Carbs: 13%

Deviled Eggs (7 Variations)

30-MINUTE **GLUTEN-FREE** **NUT-FREE** **VEGETARIAN (CLASSIC AND MEXICAN-STYLE VARIATIONS)**

This twist on deviled eggs should not be called "deviled" at all because they aren't very spicy. If you're the type to add hot sauce to everything, then the name can stay. Otherwise, think of these as stuffed eggs.

SERVES 1
PREP TIME: 10 MINUTES
COOK TIME: 10 MINUTES

FOR ALL VARIATIONS

2 large eggs

FOR CLASSIC VARIATION

1 large egg yolk

2 tablespoons minced scallions, white and green parts

½ teaspoon spicy mustard

½ tablespoon olive or avocado oil

1 teaspoon salt

1 teaspoon freshly ground black pepper

1. Bring a small pot of water to a boil over high heat. Using a slotted spoon, put the eggs in the water. Cook for about 10 minutes.

2. Meanwhile, fill a medium bowl with water and ice.

3. While the eggs are cooking, prep the remaining ingredients, depending on which variety of deviled eggs you're making.

4. When the eggs are finished cooking, use a slotted spoon to transfer them from the pot to the ice bath to cool.

5. When the eggs are cool, carefully peel them and slice them in half lengthwise. Scoop out the egg yolks, and put them in a mixing bowl.

6. Add the ingredients for the variation you're making and mix together well.

7. Using a small spoon, fill each egg-white cavity with the mixture and devour!

PER SERVING (2 EGGS): Calories: 122; Total Fat: 10g; Protein: 7g; Total Carbs: 1g; Fiber: 0g; Net Carbs: 1g
MACROS: Fat: 74% / Protein: 23% / Carbs: 3%

CONTINUED >>

FOR SARDINE OR SALMON VARIATION

1 large egg yolk

½ (4.25-ounce) can water- or olive oil–packed sardines or salmon

2 cherry tomatoes, diced

¼ small avocado, pitted, peeled, and mashed (if using fish packed in water)

½ teaspoon Dijon mustard

FOR SPICY TUNA VARIATION

1 large egg yolk

2 ounces sushi-grade ahi tuna

½ teaspoon toasted sesame oil

½ teaspoon spicy mustard

1 teaspoon tamari or coconut aminos

Sesame seeds, for garnish

FOR GROUND BEEF VARIATION

1 large egg yolk

2 ounces cooked 80% lean ground beef

¼ small avocado, pitted, peeled, and mashed

Salt

Freshly ground black pepper

FOR CHICKEN VARIATION

1 large egg yolk

2 ounces cooked ground or diced chicken

2 teaspoons diced tomatoes

¼ small avocado, pitted, peeled, and mashed, or ½ tablespoon olive or avocado oil

1 teaspoon garlic powder

1 teaspoon onion powder

Salt

Freshly ground black pepper

Sugar-free hot sauce (optional)

FOR MEXICAN-STYLE VARIATION

1 large egg yolk

¼ small avocado, pitted, peeled, and mashed

1 tablespoon salsa

Salt

Freshly ground black pepper

FOR THANKSGIVING-STYLE VARIATION

1 large egg yolk

2 tablespoons mashed or pureed pumpkin or butternut squash

2 tablespoons diced, roasted Brussels sprouts

2 ounces diced, cooked turkey

1 or 2 fresh cranberries, for topping (optional)

SARDINE OR SALMON PER SERVING: Calories: 179; Total Fat: 11g; Protein: 14g; Total Carbs: 6g; Fiber: 2g; Net Carbs: 4g
MACROS: Fat: 55% / Protein: 31% / Carbs: 14%

SPICY TUNA PER SERVING: Calories: 155; Total Fat: 10g; Protein: 15g; Total Carbs: 1g; Fiber: 0g; Net Carbs: 1g
MACROS: Fat: 60% / Protein: 37% / Carbs: 3%

GROUND BEEF PER SERVING: Calories: 248; Total Fat: 16g; Protein: 13g; Total Carbs: 3g; Fiber: 2g; Net Carbs: 1g
MACROS: Fat: 60% / Protein: 37% / Carbs: 3%

CHICKEN PER SERVING: Calories: 180; Total Fat: 12g; Protein: 15g; Total Carbs: 3g; Fiber: 1g; Net Carbs: 2g
MACROS: Fat: 60% / Protein: 33% / Carbs: 7%

MEXICAN-STYLE PER SERVING: Calories: 147; Total Fat: 11g; Protein: 8g; Total Carbs: 4g; Fiber: 2g; Net Carbs: 2g
MACROS: Fat: 68% / Protein: 22% / Carbs: 10%

THANKSGIVING-STYLE PER SERVING: Calories: 144; Total Fat: 8g; Protein: 16g; Total Carbs: 3g; Fiber: 1g; Net Carbs: 2g
MACROS: Fat: 48% / Protein: 45% / Carbs: 7%

TIP: You can find roasted Brussels sprouts at places like Trader Joe's. Look for pureed pumpkin and butternut squash in the canned vegetable aisle.

TIP: Use Keto Mayonnaise (page 186) instead of olive oil or avocado for any of these variations.

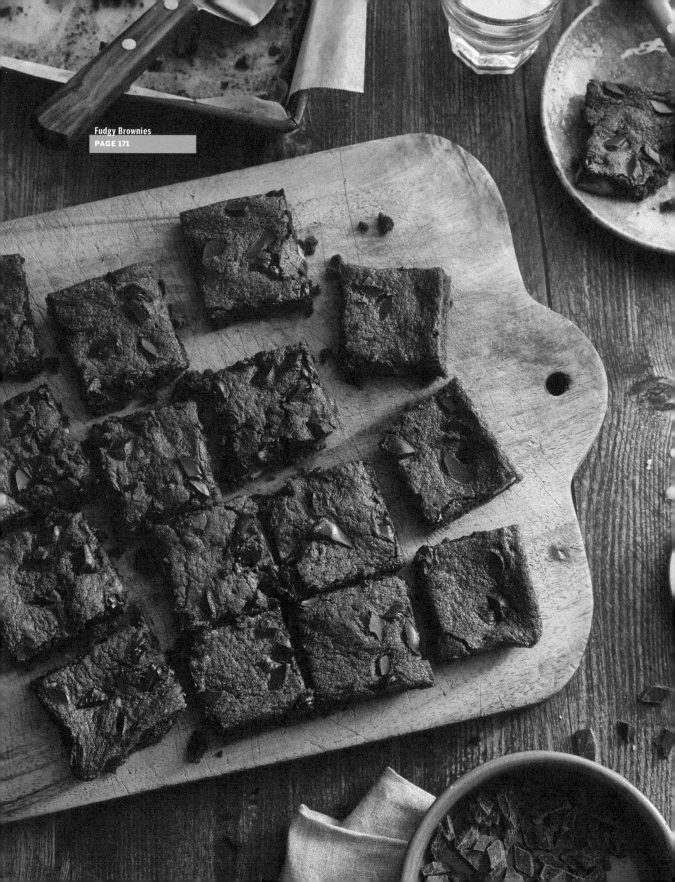

Fudgy Brownies
PAGE 171

Desserts

Mug Cake Three Ways

30-MINUTE **GLUTEN-FREE** **VEGETARIAN**

These recipes use almond milk, flavored extracts, and powders to avoid dry, eggy mug cakes. Be sure to mix the ingredients in a bowl before putting them in the mug to avoid ingredients clumping in the mug. If you want icing, use whipped heavy cream or coconut cream.

SERVES 1
PREP TIME: 10 MINUTES
COOK TIME: 1 MINUTE

FOR ALL MUG CAKES

3 tablespoons almond flour

1 large egg, beaten

1 tablespoon butter, melted and cooled

½ teaspoon baking powder

FOR A VANILLA MUG CAKE

1½ tablespoons plus 2 teaspoons erythritol

1 tablespoon coconut flour

⅛ teaspoon ground cinnamon

1 tablespoon unsweetened vanilla almond milk

1½ teaspoons vanilla extract

Nonstick cooking spray

FOR A CHOCOLATE MUG CAKE

½ tablespoon unsweetened cocoa powder

1 tablespoon erythritol

1 tablespoon unsweetened vanilla almond milk

Nonstick cooking spray

FOR A LEMON MUG CAKE

1½ tablespoons plus 1 teaspoon erythritol

1 tablespoon coconut flour

1 tablespoon unsweetened vanilla almond milk

1 teaspoon grated lemon zest

1 teaspoon lemon extract

Nonstick cooking spray

1. In a medium bowl, combine the almond flour, beaten egg, butter, and baking powder. Whisk until just mixed.

2. To the same bowl, add all the ingredients for your chosen mug cake (except the cooking spray) and whisk again.

3. Spray a large, microwave-safe mug with cooking spray and pour in the batter.

4. Microwave on high for 60 seconds. If the edges are pulling away from the sides of the mug, but the middle looks slightly underdone, the mug cake is done. If not, cook it in 15-second intervals until done.

5. Let the mug cake cool for 1 to 2 minutes. Remove it with a spatula or butter knife or eat it straight out of the mug.

PER SERVING (1 VANILLA MUG CAKE): Calories: 352; Total Fat: 29g; Protein: 12g; Total Carbs: 38g; Fiber: 5g; Net Carbs: 33g
MACROS: Fat: 74% / Protein: 14% / Carbs: 12%

PER SERVING (1 CHOCOLATE MUG CAKE): Calories: 334; Total Fat: 29g; Protein: 14g; Total Carbs: 25g; Fiber: 7g; Net Carbs: 18g
MACROS: Fat: 78% / Protein: 17% / Carbs: 5%

PER SERVING (1 LEMON MUG CAKE): Calories: 334; Total Fat: 29g; Protein: 12g; Total Carbs: 34g; Fiber: 5g; Net Carbs: 29g
MACROS: Fat: 78% / Protein: 14% / Carbs: 8%

Zucchini Chocolate Bread

DAIRY-FREE **GLUTEN-FREE** **VEGETARIAN**

Made with shredded zucchini and unsweetened cocoa powder, this bread is not overly sweet but will still satisfy your sweet tooth. Also, the fiber in the loaf will keep you feeling full for longer and aid the digestive process.

MAKES 1 (9-INCH) LOAF
PREP TIME: 15 MINUTES
COOK TIME: 1 HOUR

½ cup coconut oil, melted, plus more for greasing

1 cup almond flour

1 cup erythritol

½ cup coconut flour

¼ cup unsweetened cocoa powder

1½ teaspoons baking powder

1 teaspoon ground cinnamon

½ teaspoon baking soda

¼ teaspoon salt

4 large eggs

2 teaspoons vanilla extract

2 cups finely grated zucchini

1. Preheat the oven to 350°F. Lightly grease a 9-by-4-inch loaf pan with coconut oil.

2. In a large bowl, stir together the almond flour, erythritol, coconut flour, cocoa powder, baking powder, cinnamon, baking soda, and salt, until well blended.

3. In a medium bowl, whisk the eggs, coconut oil, and vanilla until mixed.

4. Add the wet ingredients to the dry ingredients and stir until just combined. Stir in the zucchini.

5. Spoon the batter into the prepared loaf pan and bake until a toothpick inserted into the center comes out clean, about 1 hour.

6. Let the bread cool completely before serving. Store leftovers wrapped in the refrigerator for up to 4 days or in the freezer for up to 1 month.

PER SERVING (⅛ RECIPE): Calories: 286; Total Fat: 22g; Protein: 8g; Total Carbs: 14g; Fiber: 8g; Net Carbs: 6g
MACROS: Fat: 67% / Protein: 14% / Carbs: 19%

Fudgy Brownies

GLUTEN-FREE

There are cakey brownies, and there are fudgy brownies. These are the latter. The key to a fudgy brownie is to not overmix the batter. (That makes them cakey.) If you're feeling extra indulgent, swap the vanilla extract for hazelnut to create a Nutella-tasting treat.

MAKES 16 BROWNIES
PREP TIME: 15 MINUTES
COOK TIME: 20 MINUTES

5 tablespoons butter, at room temperature

⅔ cup erythritol

1 cup almond flour

⅓ cup unsweetened cocoa powder

1 teaspoon baking powder

¼ teaspoon sea salt

2 large eggs, at room temperature

1 teaspoon vanilla extract

3 tablespoons unsweetened vanilla almond milk

½ cup sugar-free chocolate chunks or chopped walnuts, divided

1. Preheat the oven to 350°F. Line an 8-by-8-inch baking dish with parchment paper.

2. In a large bowl, beat together the butter and erythritol until the sweetener dissolves.

3. In another large bowl, whisk together the flour, cocoa powder, baking powder, and salt.

4. Beat half of the dry mixture into the butter, then beat in 1 egg. Repeat with the remaining dry mix and the remaining egg.

5. Beat in the vanilla and then the almond milk. As soon as the almond milk incorporates, stop mixing the batter. It should appear thinner than a cookie batter, resembling a boxed cake mix. Gently fold in half the chocolate chips.

6. Pour the mixture into the prepared dish and top evenly with the remaining chocolate chips.

CONTINUED >>

7. Bake for 20 minutes or until the top is set but the center is still fudgy. Don't over-bake these; if your oven runs hot, start checking them at 18 minutes.

8. Let the brownies cool at room tempera-ture for at least 30 minutes before slicing and serving. Store leftovers in an airtight container or sealed plastic bag at room temperature for up to 6 days.

PER SERVING (1 BROWNIE): Calories: 106; Total Fat: 10g; Protein: 3g; Total Carbs: 14g; Fiber: 3g; Net Carbs: 11g
MACROS: Fat: 85% / Protein: 11% / Carbs: 4%

Chocolate Almond Fudge

5-INGREDIENT **GLUTEN-FREE** **VEGAN**

Ready to have the best fudge ever? Keep a supply of this fudge in the freezer for when you're in the mood for something both sweet and salty.

MAKE 12 SQUARES
PREP TIME: 5 MINUTES, PLUS 30 MINUTES TO FREEZE

1 cup coconut oil

¼ cup unsweetened cocoa powder

½ teaspoon stevia or 4 drops liquid stevia extract

1 teaspoon vanilla extract

¼ cup almond butter

¼ teaspoon salt

1. Line a 5-inch square baking dish with parchment paper overhanging the sides.

2. In a small saucepan, melt the coconut oil over low heat. Add the cocoa powder and stevia, stirring until completely smooth. Remove from the heat and stir in the vanilla.

3. Taste and add additional stevia if you prefer more sweetness.

4. Pour the mixture into the prepared dish. Use a spoon to swirl the almond butter over the top, then sprinkle with the salt.

5. Freeze for 30 minutes or until solid and firm.

6. Using the parchment paper as handles, carefully transfer the fudge to a cutting board. Cut the fudge into squares and serve. Store leftovers in a sealed container in the freezer.

PER SERVING (1 SQUARE): Calories: 235; Total Fat: 23g; Protein: 2g; Total Carbs: 5g; Fiber: 2g; Net Carbs: 3g
MACROS: Fat: 88% / Protein: 4% / Carbs: 8%

Buttercream Pudding "Fluff"

30-MINUTE **GLUTEN-FREE**

This dessert is nicknamed "fluff," but it's a lot like icing, and you can make it in infinite flavors. The base of the recipe is butter and cream cheese. Whatever else you want to add is up to you. Try berries, nuts, sugar-free chocolate chips, and different flavorings—it's especially good with some homemade, sugar-free whipped cream on top. Just be sure to add the additional carbs to your total.

MAKES 3¹⁄₃ CUPS
PREP TIME: 10 MINUTES

2½ (8-ounce) packages full-fat cream cheese, at room temperature

8 tablespoons (1 stick) butter

1 tablespoon ground cinnamon

1 teaspoon vanilla extract

1 squeeze liquid stevia extract

½ cup chopped pecans

2 tablespoons sugar-free brown sugar (see tip)

1. In a large bowl, use a handheld electric mixer on high speed to whip together the cream cheese, butter, cinnamon, vanilla, and stevia.

2. Gently fold in the pecans and brown sugar until just incorporated.

3. Pour the mixture into a casserole or baking dish, or divide into 10 small serving bowls.

4. Store in the refrigerator until ready to serve.

TIP: Make sure your sugar-free brown sugar is a 1:1 replacement for real sugar. Swerve has a brown sugar replacement that works great. You can also add a pinch of it on top of the fluff for decoration.

PER SERVING (¹⁄₃ CUP): Calories: 329; Total Fat: 33g; Protein: 5g; Total Carbs: 3g; Fiber: 1g; Net Carbs: 2g
MACROS: Fat: 90% / Protein: 6% / Carbs: 4%

Strawberries and Cream Cake

30-MINUTE **GLUTEN-FREE** **VEGETARIAN**

Make this sweet, creamy cake in the spring when plump strawberries arrive at the market. It makes for the perfect dessert, of course, but you can also enjoy it for breakfast when you want something indulgent with which to start the day.

SERVES 1
PREP TIME: 10 MINUTES
COOK TIME: 5 MINUTES

2 large eggs

¼ cup low- to zero-carb vanilla syrup (see tip)

2 tablespoons ghee, melted and cooled

2 tablespoons full-fat cream cheese, at room temperature

¼ cup almond flour

4 strawberries, hulled and cut into chunks

¼ cup sugar-free whipped cream

1. In a blender, combine the eggs, vanilla syrup, ghee, and cream cheese. Blend until well mixed. Scrape the mixture into a small, microwave-safe bowl.

2. Stir in the almond flour, then the strawberries.

3. Microwave on high for 4 minutes until risen.

4. Let the cake cool for a minute, then top it with the whipped cream.

TIP: The vanilla sweetener makes all the difference in this recipe. You can find it online and at specialty grocery stores. Look for the brands Torani (made with Splenda) and Monin (made with Splenda and erythritol).

PER SERVING (ENTIRE RECIPE): Calories: 719; Total Fat: 67g; Protein: 15g; Total Carbs: 10g; Fiber: 4g; Net Carbs: 6g
MACROS: Fat: 84% / Protein: 11% / Carbs: 5%

Olive Oil Ice Cream

5-INGREDIENT | **GLUTEN-FREE** | **NUT-FREE** | **VEGETARIAN**

If you've never had olive oil ice cream before, you're in for a treat. This rich custard has a slightly savory note to it that's so much more complex than typical ice cream. Be sure to choose an olive oil variety that's light and fruity—it's worth spending the extra money for a quality olive oil for this ice cream.

MAKES 5 CUPS
PREP TIME: 10 MINUTES, PLUS 12 HOURS TO CHILL
COOK TIME: 25 MINUTES

4 large egg yolks

1/3 cup powdered sugar-free sweetener (such as stevia or monk fruit extract)

2 cups half-and-half, or 1 cup heavy whipping cream and 1 cup whole milk

1 teaspoon vanilla extract

1/8 teaspoon salt

1/4 cup extra-virgin olive oil

1. In a large bowl, whisk the egg yolks and sugar-free sweetener.

2. In a small saucepan, heat the half-and-half over medium heat until just below a boil. Remove from the heat and allow to cool slightly.

3. Slowly pour the warm half-and-half into the egg mixture, whisking constantly to avoid cooking the eggs. Return the eggs and cream to the saucepan over low heat.

4. Whisking constantly, cook until thickened, 15 to 20 minutes. Remove from the heat and stir in the vanilla and salt. Whisk in the olive oil and transfer to a glass bowl. Allow to cool, then cover, and refrigerate for at least 6 hours.

5. Using an electric mixer on medium-high speed, whip the custard until doubled in volume. Freeze for at least 6 hours before serving.

TIP: You can also prepare this recipe in an ice cream maker, if you have one.

PER SERVING (1/2 CUP): Calories: 235; Total Fat: 25g; Protein: 23g; Total Carbs: 2g; Fiber: 0g, Net Carbs: 2g
MACROS: Fat: 94% / Protein: 4% / Carbs: 2%

Crustless Lemon Cheesecake

GLUTEN-FREE **NUT-FREE**

Unbaked cheesecakes are often almost bouncy in their texture because they contain too much gelatin for the ingredient ratio, but this recipe fixes that. This lemon cheesecake still has the slightly grainy texture of cream cheese instead of that of creamy Jell-O. You can use sheet gelatin instead of granules, but getting the substitution ratio correct is difficult; it's about three sheets to a packet.

MAKES 4 SMALL CHEESECAKES
PREP TIME: 15 MINUTES, PLUS 1 HOUR TO SET

1 (7g) package plain gelatin

¼ cup heavy (whipping) cream

8 ounces full-fat cream cheese, at room temperature

2 tablespoons freshly squeezed lemon juice

1 teaspoon stevia

1 teaspoon vanilla extract

1. In a small bowl, sprinkle the gelatin over the heavy cream. Set aside for 10 minutes.

2. In a large bowl, beat the cream cheese with a handheld electric mixer on high speed until smooth and fluffy, about 4 minutes.

3. Beat in the lemon juice, stevia, and vanilla, scraping down the sides of the bowl at least once. Add the heavy cream mixture to the large bowl and beat to blend.

4. Spoon the lemon cheesecake mixture into four small serving dishes and chill until set, about 1 hour. Serve.

PER SERVING (1 CHEESECAKE): Calories: 235; Total Fat: 23g; Protein: 7g; Total Carbs: 2g; Fiber: 0g; Net Carbs: 2g
MACROS: Fat: 84% / Protein: 12% / Carbs: 4%

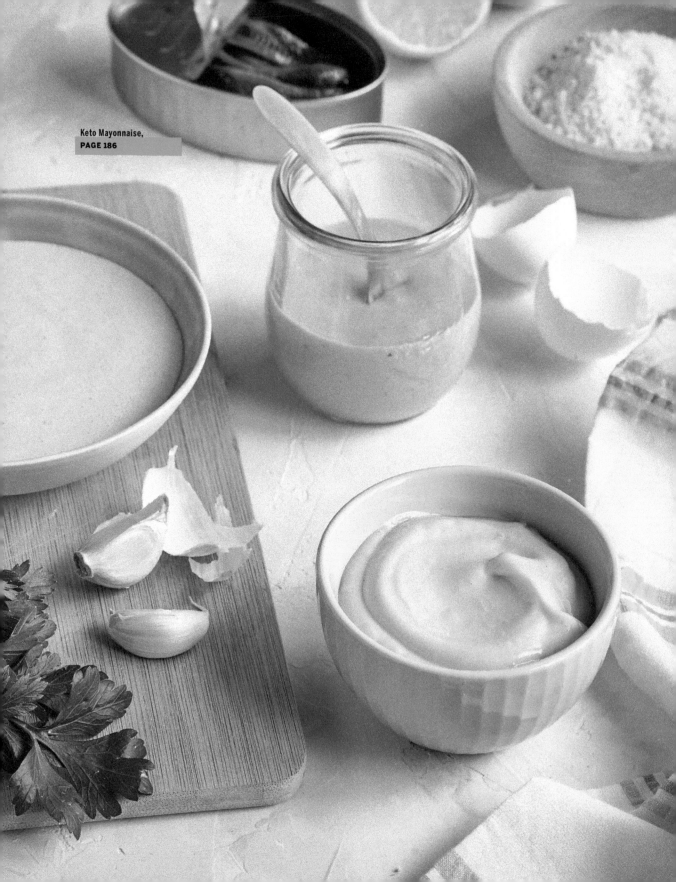

Keto Mayonnaise,
PAGE 186

Staples

Basic Broth

ONE POT **GLUTEN-FREE** **NUT-FREE** **VEGAN**

Broth takes a little effort to make, but it's well worth it. After all, you can never be sure about the additives and ingredients in store-bought soups. For a set-it-and-forget-it method, use a slow cooker instead of a pot on the stove. Simply toss the ingredients inside the slow cooker and fill with water until it reaches 1½ inches from the top. Cover and cook the broth on low for 10 to 12 hours, strain out the solids, cool, and store. Now you have a simple option for an electrolyte boost or a delicious base for any soup.

MAKES 8 CUPS
PREP TIME: 15 MINUTES
COOK TIME: 2 TO 3 HOURS

3 celery stalks with greens, roughly chopped

2 carrots, roughly chopped

1 medium yellow onion, peeled and quartered

½ cup chopped fresh parsley

4 garlic cloves, crushed

4 thyme sprigs

2 bay leaves

½ teaspoon black peppercorns

½ teaspoon salt

8 cups water

1. In a large stockpot, combine the celery, carrots, onion, parsley, garlic, thyme, bay leaves, peppercorns, and salt.

2. Pour in the water, cover, and bring to a boil. Reduce the heat to low and simmer gently for 2 to 3 hours.

3. Strain the broth through a fine-mesh sieve and discard the solids.

4. Store the broth in sealed containers in the refrigerator for up to 5 days or in the freezer for up to 1 month.

BEEF BROTH VARIATION

Add 2 to 3 pounds of beef bones (beef marrow, knuckle bones, ribs, and any other bones) and 2 tablespoons of apple cider vinegar in step 1 of the Basic Broth recipe and enough water to cover the extra ingredients. Simmer, scooping off any accumulating foam, for 6 to 7 hours. (Don't scoop if using a slow cooker.) Strain the broth through a fine-mesh sieve, discarding the solids. After cooling, store the broth in sealed containers in the refrigerator for up to 1 week or in the freezer for up to 3 months. Makes 8 cups.

CHICKEN BROTH VARIATION

Add 2 chicken carcasses and 2 tablespoons of apple cider vinegar in step 1 of the Basic Broth recipe and enough water to cover the extra ingredients. Simmer, scooping off any accumulating foam, for 4 to 5 hours. (Don't scoop if using a slow cooker.) Strain the broth through a fine-mesh sieve, discarding the solids. After cooling, store the broth in sealed containers in the refrigerator for up to 1 week or in the freezer for up to 3 months. Makes 8 cups.

FISH BROTH VARIATION

Add 3 to 4 pounds of fish bones and heads to the Basic Broth recipe and enough water to cover the extra ingredients. Simmer for 1 hour and then strain the broth through a fine-mesh sieve, discarding the solids. After cooling, store the broth in sealed containers in the refrigerator for up to 1 week or in the freezer for up to 3 months. Makes 8 cups.

VEGETABLE BROTH PER SERVING (1 CUP): Calories: 24; Total Fat: 0g; Protein: 2g; Total Carbs: 4g; Fiber: 0g; Net Carbs: 4g
MACROS: Fat: 2% / Protein: 32% / Carbs: 66%

BEEF BROTH PER SERVING (1 CUP): Calories: 42; Total Fat: 1g; Protein: 8g; Total Carbs: 0g; Fiber: 0g; Net Carbs: 0g
MACROS: Fat: 20% / Protein: 76% / Carbs: 4%

CHICKEN BROTH PER SERVING (1 CUP): Calories: 38; Total Fat: 0g; Protein: 9g; Total Carbs: 0g; Fiber: 0g; Net Carbs: 0g
MACROS: Fat: 5% / Protein: 94% / Carbs: 1%

FISH BROTH PER SERVING (1 CUP): Calories: 34; Total Fat: 1g; Protein: 7g; Total Carbs: 0g; Fiber: 0g; Net Carbs: 0g
MACROS: Fat: 26% / Protein: 72% / Carbs: 2%

90-Second Bread

5-INGREDIENT **30-MINUTE** **GLUTEN-FREE** **VEGETARIAN**

This bread is incredibly versatile, taking on different flavor profiles when various fats and seasonings are used. The base recipe produces a traditional bread flavor that is best used anytime you're craving the comfort of sliced white bread. You can easily add up to 1 tablespoon of erythritol to make this bread sweet.

SERVES 1
PREP TIME: 3 MINUTES
**COOK TIME: 1 MINUTE,
30 SECONDS**

1 large egg

3 tablespoons almond flour

1 tablespoon melted butter

¼ teaspoon baking powder

Pinch sea salt

Nonstick cooking spray

1. In a small bowl, beat the egg with a fork or whisk. Whisk in the almond flour, butter, baking powder, and salt until completely combined.

2. Spray the inside of a large coffee mug with cooking spray.

3. Pour the mixture into the mug and microwave for 90 seconds.

4. Let the bread cool slightly and then remove it from the mug. It should slide right out.

5. Slice the bread in half and either enjoy as is, with your preferred toppings, or toasted for some extra crunch.

PER SERVING (1 BREAD): Calories: 300; Total Fat: 27g; Protein: 11g; Total Carbs: 5g; Fiber: 2g; Net Carbs: 3g
MACROS: Fat: 79%; Protein: 14%; Carbs: 7%

Taco Seasoning

30-MINUTE | ONE BOWL | GLUTEN-FREE | NUT-FREE | VEGAN

Give any meal some Mexican-inspired flair with this super easy taco seasoning. Mix it into ground beef or rub it onto chicken, steak, or shrimp. It also tastes great mixed into sour cream or melted cheese for a quick dip.

MAKES ½ CUP
PREP TIME: 5 MINUTES

4 tablespoons ground cumin

1 tablespoon garlic powder

1 tablespoon chili powder

1 tablespoon onion powder

2 teaspoons dried oregano

2 teaspoons smoked paprika

In a sealable container, combine the cumin, garlic powder, chili powder, onion powder, oregano, and paprika. Store at room temperature for up to 6 months.

PER SERVING (1 TABLESPOON): Calories: 29; Total Fat: 1g; Protein: 1g; Total Carbs: 4g; Fiber: 1g; Net Carbs: 3g
MACROS: Fat: 31%; Protein: 14%; Carbs: 55%

Guacamole

Holy guacamole! Here is my spin on a classic. Whether you eat it with a spoon, use it as a dip, or pile it high on a taco salad, you can't go wrong with guacamole.

MAKES 1 CUP
PREP TIME: 15 MINUTES

1 avocado, pitted and peeled

¼ medium red onion, diced

1 teaspoon freshly squeezed lime juice

¼ tablespoon ground cumin

¼ tablespoon garlic powder

1 teaspoon minced fresh cilantro (optional)

Salt

1. Put the avocado in a medium bowl. With a fork, mash to your preferred consistency.

2. Add the onion, lime juice, cumin, garlic powder, and cilantro (if using). Mix well.

3. Season with salt to taste. Serve immediately.

PER SERVING (½ CUP): Calories: 165; Total Fat: 13g; Protein: 2g; Total Carbs: 10g; Fiber: 6g; Net Carbs: 4g
MACROS: Fat: 71% / Protein: 5% / Carbs: 24%

Butternut Squash "Cheese" Sauce

`30-MINUTE` `GLUTEN-FREE` `NUT-FREE` `VEGAN`

Although cheese is absolutely acceptable on the keto diet, this dairy-free sauce is a great option for those who need to avoid dairy or when you simply want to change things up. Pour this "cheese" sauce over vegetable noodles or drizzle it over grilled chicken. Or make it in bulk and freeze it in ice cube trays for future portion-size use.

MAKES 2 CUPS
PREP TIME: 10 MINUTES
COOK TIME: 10 MINUTES

1 tablespoon coconut oil

2 cups frozen, cubed butternut squash

2 tablespoons nutritional yeast

1 tablespoon tahini

1 teaspoon garlic powder

½ teaspoon onion powder

½ teaspoon smoked paprika

¼ teaspoon salt

¼ teaspoon freshly ground black pepper

1. In a shallow sauté pan, heat the coconut oil over medium-high heat. When it shimmers, add the frozen butternut squash and cook until it is no longer frozen and the liquid in the pan has evaporated, 5 to 8 minutes.

2. Transfer the cooked squash to a blender; add the nutritional yeast, tahini, garlic powder, onion powder, paprika, salt, and pepper. Blend until completely smooth. Serve immediately.

TIP: Try using pumpkin in this recipe instead of butternut squash.

PER SERVING (⅓ CUP): Calories: 64; Total Fat: 4g; Protein: 3g; Total Carbs: 7g; Fiber: 1g; Net Carbs: 6g
MACROS: Fat: 54% / Protein: 7% / Carbs: 39%

Keto Mayonnaise

5-INGREDIENT | **30-MINUTE** | **ONE BOWL** | **DAIRY-FREE** | **GLUTEN-FREE** | **NUT-FREE** | **VEGETARIAN**

This mayonnaise is simple to make and will keep for up to a week in the refrigerator. It makes for a guilt-free addition to just about any dish. Incorporating mayonnaise into your meal is a great way to reach your fat goals for the day.

MAKES ABOUT 2 CUPS
PREP TIME: 10 MINUTES

2 large egg yolks, at room temperature

2 tablespoons freshly squeezed lemon juice

1 tablespoon apple cider vinegar

1 teaspoon salt

1 teaspoon Dijon mustard

1½ cups olive oil or avocado oil

1. In a food processor, combine the yolks, lemon juice, vinegar, salt, and mustard, and blend for about 30 seconds or until well combined.

2. With the food processor on high speed, slowly drizzle in the oil in a thin stream until the mixture thickens.

3. Store in a glass jar or airtight container in the refrigerator for up to 1 week.

TIP: To make this recipe vegan, replace the egg yolks with 2 tablespoons of coconut oil.

PER SERVING (2 TABLESPOONS): Calories: 187; Total Fat: 21g; Protein: 0g; Total Carbs: 0g; Fiber: 0g; Net Carbs: 0g
MACROS: Fat: 99% / Protein: 1% / Carbs: 0%

Ranch Dressing

30-MINUTE ONE BOWL GLUTEN-FREE NUT-FREE VEGETARIAN

This classic dressing is great as a dip for veggies and breaded meats, and of course as a dressing for green salads. It's really easy to make at home, which helps you cut down on the amount of preservatives you consume. If you want, make a big batch of the spice mix so it's ready to go when you need it (it's also a great way to season meat before grilling).

MAKES ABOUT 1½ CUPS
PREP TIME: 5 MINUTES

1 cup Keto Mayonnaise (page 186) or store-bought mayonnaise

½ cup sour cream

1½ teaspoons dried chives

1 teaspoon mustard powder

½ teaspoon dried dill

½ teaspoon celery seed

½ teaspoon onion powder

½ teaspoon garlic powder

Salt

Freshly ground black pepper

In a medium bowl, combine the mayonnaise, sour cream, chives, mustard powder, dill, celery seed, onion powder, and garlic powder. Season with salt and pepper to taste. Stir well to combine, then store in an airtight container in the refrigerator for up to 1 week.

PER SERVING (2 TABLESPOONS): Calories: 43; Total Fat: 3g; Protein: 1g; Total Carbs: 3g; Fiber: 1g; Net Carbs: 2g
MACROS: Fat: 63% / Protein: 9% / Carbs: 28%

Avocado-Kale Pesto

30-MINUTE | **ONE BOWL** | **GLUTEN-FREE** | **VEGAN**

The secret to this pesto? Freshly squeezed lemon juice. This special ingredient prevents the avocado puree from oxidizing and turning a dull gray. Lemons are also a good source of vitamin C and the antioxidant limonene.

MAKES 2 CUPS
PREP TIME: 15 MINUTES

1 avocado, peeled, pitted, and diced

1 cup chopped kale

½ cup fresh basil leaves

½ cup pine nuts

3 garlic cloves, peeled

1 tablespoon freshly squeezed lemon juice

2 teaspoons nutritional yeast

¼ cup extra-virgin olive oil

Sea salt

1. In a food processor, combine the avocado, kale, basil, pine nuts, garlic, lemon juice, and nutritional yeast. Pulse until finely chopped, about 2 minutes.

2. With the food processor running, drizzle the olive oil into the pesto until a thick paste forms, stopping to scrape down the sides at least once. Season with salt to taste.

3. Store the pesto in a sealed container in the refrigerator for up to 1 week.

TIP: Pesto freezes well, so whip up a batch and freeze for future use. Pop out a pesto cube (if using ice cube trays) and drop into your soup for an instant hit of flavor.

PER SERVING (2 TABLESPOONS): Calories: 92; Total Fat: 8g; Protein: 2g; Total Carbs: 3g; Fiber: 1g; Net Carbs: 2g
MACROS: Fat: 78% / Protein: 9% / Carbs: 13%

Tahini Goddess Dressing

5-INGREDIENT **30-MINUTE** **ONE BOWL** **GLUTEN-FREE** **NUT-FREE** **VEGAN**

Tahini, a Middle Eastern paste made with sesame seeds, is often used to flavor hummus and baba ghanoush. It is highly nutritious and can boost bone cell growth. The healthy fats contained in tahini also support optimal brain function.

MAKES 1 CUP
PREP TIME: 5 MINUTES

¼ cup water

Juice of 1 large or 2 small lemons

3 tablespoons raw tahini

½ teaspoon smoked paprika

⅛ teaspoon ground cayenne pepper (optional)

Sea salt

Freshly ground black pepper

1. In a medium bowl, whisk the water, lemon juice, and tahini until well blended.

2. Add the paprika and cayenne (if using), and season with salt and pepper. Mix until well combined.

3. Store the dressing in a sealed container in the pantry for up to 6 months. In the refrigerator, it will last for up to 1 year.

TIP: If you prefer a less tart flavor, add a drop or two of liquid stevia to offset the lemon juice.

PER SERVING (2 TABLESPOONS): Calories: 40; Total Fat: 3g; Protein: 1g; Total Carbs: 2g; Fiber: 1g; Net Carbs: 1g
MACROS: Fat: 68% / Protein: 10% / Carbs: 22%

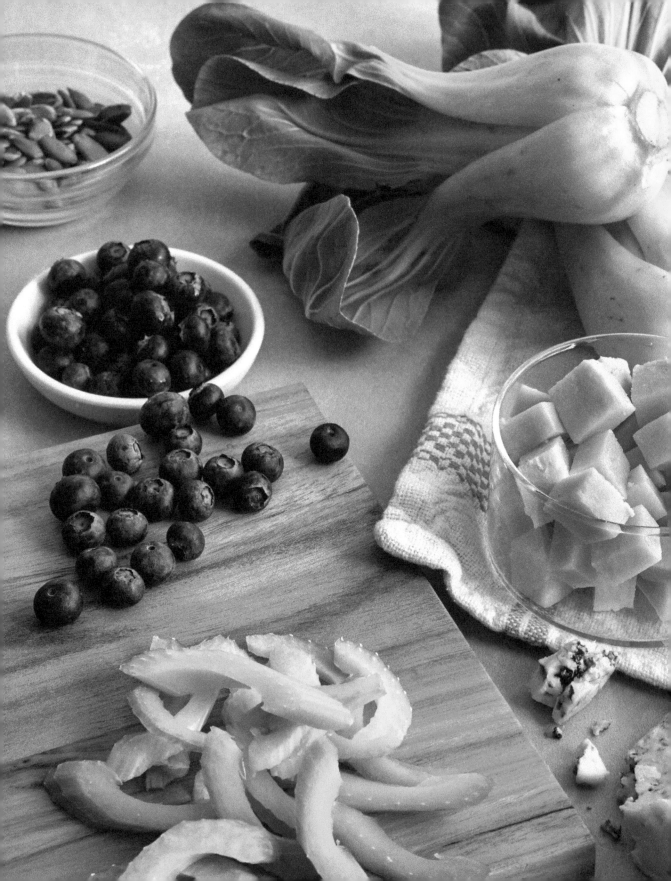

MEASUREMENT CONVERSIONS

VOLUME EQUIVALENTS	U.S. STANDARD	U.S. STANDARD (OUNCES)	METRIC (APPROXIMATE)
LIQUID	2 tablespoons	1 fl. oz.	30 mL
	¼ cup	2 fl. oz.	60 mL
	½ cup	4 fl. oz.	120 mL
	1 cup	8 fl. oz.	240 mL
	1½ cups	12 fl. oz.	355 mL
	2 cups or 1 pint	16 fl. oz.	475 mL
	4 cups or 1 quart	32 fl. oz.	1 L
	1 gallon	128 fl. oz.	4 L
DRY	⅛ teaspoon	—	0.5 mL
	¼ teaspoon	—	1 mL
	½ teaspoon	—	2 mL
	¾ teaspoon	—	4 mL
	1 teaspoon	—	5 mL
	1 tablespoon	—	15 mL
	¼ cup	—	59 mL
	⅓ cup	—	79 mL
	½ cup	—	118 mL
	⅔ cup	—	156 mL
	¾ cup	—	177 mL
	1 cup	—	235 mL
	2 cups or 1 pint	—	475 mL
	3 cups	—	700 mL
	4 cups or 1 quart	—	1 L
	½ gallon	—	2 L
	1 gallon	—	4 L

OVEN TEMPERATURES

FAHRENHEIT	CELSIUS (APPROXIMATE)
250°F	120°C
300°F	150°C
325°F	165°C
350°F	180°C
375°F	190°C
400°F	200°C
425°F	220°C
450°F	230°C

WEIGHT EQUIVALENTS

U.S. STANDARD	METRIC (APPROXIMATE)
½ ounce	15 g
1 ounce	30 g
2 ounces	60 g
4 ounces	115 g
8 ounces	225 g
12 ounces	340 g
16 ounces or 1 pound	455 g

INDEX